INSIDE THE BOX

INSIDE THE BOX

HOW CROSSFIT® SHREDDED THE RULES, STRIPPED DOWN THE GYM, AND REBUILT MY BODY

T.J. MURPHY

VELO press

Boulder, Colorado

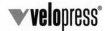

3002 Sterling Circle, Suite 100
Boulder, Colorado 80301-2338 USA
(303) 440-0601 · Fax (303) 444-6788 · E-mail velopress@competitorgroup.com

Distributed in the United States and Canada by Ingram Publisher Services

A Cataloging-in-Publication record for this book is available from the Library of Congress.
ISBN 978-1-934030-90-5

For information on purchasing VeloPress books, please call (800) 811-4210 ext. 2138 or visit
www.velopress.com.

Cover design by *the*BookDesigners
Cover photograph by Nick Rudnicki
Interior design by Erin Johnson
Interior photographs by Robert Murphy, pp. 7, 19, 37, 57, 73, 101, and 115; Scott Draper, pp. 89, 135,
and 181; and Caroline Treadway, p. 46 and all photographs in the exercise glossary

Text set in Neuton

12   13   14   /   10   9   8   7   6   5   4   3   2   1

To the coaches and athletes of CrossFit Elysium,
for their friendship and constant inspiration

CONTENTS

ACKNOWLEDGMENTS

I'd like to thank the coaches and athletes I had the pleasure of meeting in the months I was getting acquainted with the sport at the following boxes: CrossFit Cedar Rapids, CrossFit Invictus, CrossFit NYC, CrossFit Southie, CrossFit Bloomington, CrossFit East Village, and CrossFit Santa Cruz Central. I'd particularly like to thank Brian MacKenzie, Kelly and Juliet Starrett, Carl Paoli, Todd Widman, Lindsey Smith, Annie Sakamoto, Dave Castro, Nicole Carroll, Gretchen Weber, and Greg Amundson—all of whom went above and beyond in helping me with this project.

I especially want to thank the staff at VeloPress for their guidance and enthusiasm in putting together this book. While I've had the pleasure of working with them over the years at Competitor Group, this was the first direct experience I'd had in seeing their passion and professionalism up close.

PROLOGUE

"IF YOU DON'T GET THOSE WEIGHTS CHANGED IN 30 SECONDS, I'M GOING TO KICK your ass."

Jesus, I thought, as I slid a green Olympic plate onto the 45-pound bar and struggled to slide the spring collar into place. I was desperate not to show it but was teetering on being completely psyched out by the lift I was about to attempt: snapping a bar loaded to 135 pounds from the ground to overhead with a single swoop of physical effort—a "snatch," it's called, a lift that's in the Olympic Games. At 135 pounds, this lift would be exactly 20 pounds more than I'd ever managed for this move. Images of total failure were playing like demons in my mind, dampening my hopes.

Take your idea of a luxury spa with chrome weights and a country-club locker room, and then imagine the complete antithesis, and you have the gym I was competing in. San Francisco CrossFit (SFCF) sits in a parking lot behind a gigantic sporting goods store in the Presidio. There are no doors, just graffiti-painted storage containers, a plastic canopy that makes violent ripping sounds when the winds hit (which is most of the time), and black rubber mats. Illumination is provided by caged utility lights. "HTFU" is scrawled on the whiteboard set up on a cinderblock wall. It's a popular acronym in the CrossFit world meaning Harden The Fuck Up. It's not just a pop phrase here at SFCF. These people work out in the dark, in the rain, and when an anomalous wet-cold wind is blowing in.

I'm here struggling with stage two of the CrossFit Open. Kelly Starrett, owner of the gym and my coach today, has already threatened to kick my ass once, during the first stage of qualifying for the CrossFit Games. He thought I was dogging it, an act he profoundly despises (I wasn't). In the end, I'd passed stage one with more than acceptable numbers to move me a step closer to the Games. Now, today, I was taking part in the Open's 2012 stage-two qualifier.

The Games comprise a three-day festival of high-intensity athletic and fitness competitions based on a globally viral training and fitness paradigm called

CrossFit that is now practiced at 4,000 gyms (and counting) around the world. The best of the best that the CrossFit Open and Regionals will identify will make it to the three-day CrossFit Games. I was an entrant for the first time, and this was the second week of a five-week competition involving thousands of CrossFit athletes from across the country, all doing the same test that I was doing right now with SFCF's co-owner and lead coach growling at me.

"Now you have 20 seconds."

I had to HTFU. In truth, I wasn't so much dogging it as I was trying to put off what seemed like inevitable humiliation, because 135 pounds might as well have been a Volkswagen, based on my prior experience with the snatch. I was loading the weights faster now, though, as I surely didn't want to get my ass kicked by a 235-pound former professional kayaker who is at least twice as strong as me.

The competition workout went like this: I had 10 minutes to get in as many lifts as possible, following this sequence:

75 pounds—30 times
135 pounds—30 times
165 pounds—30 times
210 pounds—as many times as possible

I had hoisted the 75 pounds without a problem, but I knew I'd struggle with 135. Before the day's competition was over, the 2011 CrossFit Games champion, Rich Froning Jr., would perform 98 total reps, meaning that he burned through the 75-, 135-, and 165-pound phases like a whip and then lifted 210 pounds 8 times before his 10 minutes were up. He was the only one to break 90 reps. When I first saw the workout posted, I knew the 75-pound snatches would be a breeze. But my best effort to date at a maximum snatch, just one time, had been 115 pounds. And even that wasn't pretty. When I finally did get 115 pounds over my head, after a half hour of trying, I had been elated. And in awe of those who, like Froning, made it look easy. Now I was looking at 20 pounds more than that.

The first week of the CrossFit Open had featured a timed test to see how many burpees you could do. A "burpee" starts from the standing position and entails dropping to the push-up position on the ground and then sucking your legs back underneath you and thrusting upward into a small jump. It's a basic gymnastics sort of move that is simple to do, but after you've hammered out 25 or so of them you begin to feel like an implanted defibrillator run amok. The

"12.1" workout—where you try to do as many burpees as you can in seven minutes—was a lung-scorching test that was oddly well suited to former competitive runners like me. I performed 103, after which I staggered around in a little circle in cardiopulmonary shock, as if I'd been shot in the chest. The snatch was another animal altogether—it was not tuned to the design and accustomed mechanics of a former marathoner/Ironman® guy pushing well into his forties.

So when I shook sweat from my callused hands, hook-gripped them on the 86-inch bar's roughened sections of black oxide, and crouched down to begin the first phase of the snatch with 135 pounds, I was well aware of being watched. Not only was Starrett watching me, but also a judge and several other CrossFit Open competitors, including my girlfriend, Gretchen, who was in the final heat.

I began the lift. The leap from 75 pounds to 135 was a shock. As a beginner, what you're taught to do in the snatch is to bring the bar off the ground slowly, your body weight on your heels, and about when the bar clears your knees, you perform what's called a "jump"—a vertical explosion upward, driven from the hips, that flings the weight into the air high enough that you (ideally) push against the bar and get your body under it in a deep squat. You then (ideally) have the bar and weights hoisted directly over your head with your elbows locked out, and you squat upward so that your knees lock and you're standing tall and in control of the weight, all the bones stacked up neatly under the load. Ideally. I never appreciated Olympic weight lifting events until I started doing these kinds of lifts. I now know that the best weight lifters must weave qualities like coordination, agility, speed, and strength into a seamlessly balanced movement. I used to think it was just a matter of brute power. Not true.

I jumped, and the bar came up above my waist, maybe to around the sternum. Then gravity took over, and the bar plummeted to the ground with an unforgiving clatter. The shock of the weight, magnified by the shock of such an obvious and complete failure to even come close to getting one rep, caused adrenaline to gush into my blood. I jumped up in the air and shouted, "Fuck!"

The adrenaline rush was both good and bad. I was resolute that I was going to keep trying, if only to give my anger a place to go, but it's easy to start looking like a double-bogey golfer in a sand trap, hacking away mindlessly at a sunken ball. Yet here, within my little temper tantrum, lay part of the secret to why CrossFit had become such a powerful phenomenon over the past seven years: It is structured to use the power of competition, against others and against yourself, to yield a breakthrough level of intensity.

Three attempts and three colorful outbursts later, Starrett said calmly, "This isn't working. We need a new plan." Over the next few minutes and after several more frustrated efforts, Starrett gave me steps to follow. Narrow your grip. Make sure your chest is in the correct position. Reimagine the lift so that the bar might travel a more efficient path upward.

CROSSFIT IS STRUCTURED TO USE THE POWER OF COMPETITION, AGAINST OTHERS AND AGAINST YOURSELF, TO YIELD A BREAKTHROUGH LEVEL OF INTENSITY.

"Think of throwing the bar up, over, and behind your head." He pointed to the highway overpass behind us from the parking lot. "Throw it up over that highway."

The bar inched higher on each succeeding lift, but still gravity would reach in and the weights would crash to the rubber mats. I had less than a minute left of my 10 minutes. Again, Starrett spoke calmly to me.

"We're going to get this. Just think of throwing that bar over and behind you."

There was a certain irony that Starrett was coaching me through the CF Open. I had first met him 58 weeks earlier, before Christmas in 2010, when I had limped into this same gym with the chronic knee and back injuries that had brought my life as a runner to an end. At the age of 47, not only had I lost the capacity to enjoy running, but I was having trouble just making it through the average day. Getting out of bed, sitting in an office chair, walking up and down steps—all of this had become fraught with pain. Two words, once unthinkable, had been bandied about in regard to my future: knee replacement.

In addition to being a star coach in the CrossFit universe and an expert in movement and mobility, Starrett has a doctorate in physical therapy. It was when I was at the brink of what I was sure was destined to be knee surgery that another star CrossFit coach, Brian MacKenzie, suggested I go see Starrett. The ensuing 14 months would become a long and deep look into a world that I would ordinarily have dismissed as yet another infomercial-driven exercise regimen, only in this case propped up by a cult following that, from what I could tell through the Internet, was a tattoo-mad world.

That meeting with Starrett turned out to be fortuitous. In 58 weeks he and MacKenzie had set me on a course that transformed me from a limping former runner who couldn't do 15 push-ups to one of 62,000 people competing to enter the 2012 CrossFit Games.

"You're going to get this, T.J. You've got 30 seconds."

When I looked down at the bar for what was certainly my final shot at making the lift and getting a score of 31 reps, I felt an electric shimmer course through my body. One thing the CrossFit Open offered that was similar to what I loved about running races was the chance to put fitness to a test in a situation where there's drama to be played out, a game to be played. Getting 31 as opposed to 12 or 30—or 65, for that matter—would matter little in the overall scoring of the event. I would be buried in the deep middle of the 62,000 who were competing. For the elites, it's about qualifying for the Games, but for the masses, it's those arbitrary objectives that ultimately offer the simple pleasure of personal satisfaction; reaching a new CrossFit threshold is like breaking a four-hour marathon for the first time or finishing a first triathlon. It's the satisfaction of being an athlete, as opposed to just being stuck as a spectator watching sports on TV.

So for me, in that moment, the difference between 30 and 31 was emotionally charged. Snatching 135 pounds would break my old personal record of 115 pounds. I was amped. I hopped up in the air, shaking my head as if to clear it. When I grasped the bar for what would be my final chance, butterflies in my stomach, I felt a smile crease on my face for the first time during the workout: I knew I was going to get the lift. I curled my hands onto the bar with the narrower grip Kelly had suggested, locking my thumbs underneath my fingers in the hook grip, an Olympic-lifting fundamental; crouched down; took a deep breath; and slowly began the move. With the image in my mind of catapulting the bar over my head and into the Presidio, I did the jump phase of the lift. The bar popped up one last invaluable inch higher, and I performed the turnover as quickly as possible, getting my arms and elbows underneath the bar while it was weightless. If I were better at the snatch, I would have been squatting down beneath the bar and pressing down, but I just did not yet have anywhere near that ability, and so I did what I could do—muscle the thing up into the air. This time, the last time, with five seconds left on the clock, some sort of critical point in space was passed, and instead of the bar plunging downward, it continued to rise, with an aching slowness at first, but then gaining speed. With a few seconds remaining, my elbows locked out, I had my new 135-pound personal record.

In a move that showed a complete lack of cool, I again leaped into the air, this time like a grade school Little League hero. Not cool, no, and really, a 135-pound snatch is quite modest for my weight class in the CrossFit world. But here's the thing: I leaped into the air on the very same legs and knees that I could barely step onto a curb with a year before.

This is the story of that year.

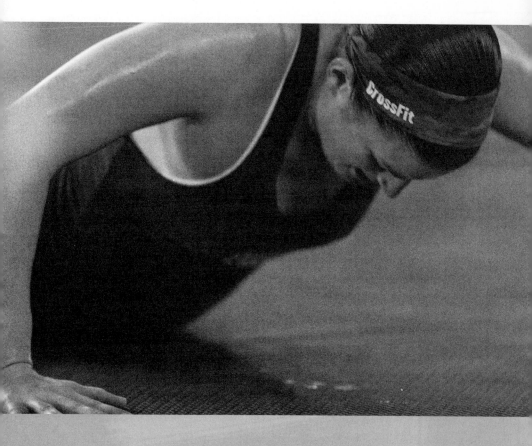

THE ENCOUNTER

THE MANY PATHS TO CROSSFIT

1

PAUL ESTRADA WAS A PERSONAL TRAINER WHO DISCOVERED CROSSFIT ON THE
Internet. After trying one of the workouts, he found himself curled up on the ground in the corner of a gym for a full seven minutes before he could stand up again. He was so hooked by the experience that he went charging into CrossFit and never looked back. Peggy Baker was in her fifties when she reluctantly followed friends into a CrossFit gym in the Boston area. A diabetic for two decades, she was overweight, sick, and getting sicker, but in a few short months she'd be in tears recounting the story of how her Type 2 diabetes had started to recede and her need for insulin shots along with it. David Bennett was in the U.S. Air Force when he was lifting some weights and saw a buddy doing a CrossFit workout on a nearby track. He was so enthralled by what he saw that he started doing CrossFit, too; he now pledges that one of his goals is to "CrossFit till death."

CrossFit has famously forged deeply dedicated believers, but perhaps most surprising of all is the astounding array of people those believers include. Anthony Kimpo does jujitsu and tried CrossFit to increase his strength. He's now as much a CrossFitter as he is a martial artist. Briana Dawn was going to school by day and working as a police dispatcher by night, eating too many of her meals at Denny's. She was 30 pounds overweight. She joined a CrossFit gym, and within a year was competing in CrossFit competitions, sleek, buff, and fit. Brian MacKenzie discovered that CrossFit helped him manage a form of boredom that, if it wasn't staved off, made him destructive, as in drinking hard, fighting, and worse. He now uses CrossFit to run 100-mile trail runs and leads a global pack of runners and triathletes through CrossFit endurance workouts. Irene Mejia was over 400 pounds, morbidly obese, and teetering on the edge of a slew of chronic diseases that come along with Type 2 diabetes when she worked up the courage to press the send button on an e-mail to a CrossFit gym asking if they'd let her try it. They said yes. Less than two years later, Irene had lost over 100 pounds and was competing in the CrossFit Games Open.

Then there's the story of Todd Widman. Widman, 25, was an officer in the U.S. Marine Corps, serving in Virginia and preparing young officers for infantry missions, when he first read about CrossFit. Widman had worked out since age 13, lifting weights through high school and his years at Oregon State. As a Marine, he had six years of dedicated bodybuilding behind him. A friend encouraged him to bypass his initial skepticism about CrossFit and check out CrossFit.com. That night, he watched the Nasty Girls video. Despite the provocative title, "Nasty Girls" is simply the name of an advanced CrossFit workout. Widman watched as three of the first-generation CrossFitters performed the workout. They were quite a mix: a former ski champion (Eva Twardokens), a former jazzercise teacher and cocktail waitress (Annie Sakamoto), and an artist who was into pottery (Nicole Carroll). Recalls Widman, "I see these little ladies doing power cleans, air squats, and muscle-ups. I wasn't sure I could do anything they were doing." In a moving display, the video zeroes in on Carroll during the final few minutes as she battles through the last round of muscle-ups and power cleans with an unmistakable look of anguish on her face.

Widman dug deeper into the site. There was no CrossFit gym near him at the time, but the web portal posted workouts on a daily basis, including some with exercises that were mysteriously named after women. Widman decided to try his hand at one called "Elizabeth"—three rounds of cleans with a 135-pound barbell and ring dips. Widman knew what a "clean" was—explosively hoisting a barbell from the ground to the position under his chin where it was racked, the first phase of an Olympic-style "clean and jerk." But then he asked, "What's a ring?" He looked through the comments section and saw that there were others asking similar questions, trying to decode the nontraditional workouts. As it turns out, "rings" were gymnastics rings, like those used for an Iron Cross. "Ring dips" were essentially what he knew to be triceps dips, a popular exercise at most commercial gyms, but done with wooden rings that hung from two straps rather than with bars or a triceps machine.

Elizabeth consisted of three rounds. In the first, he'd be doing 21 cleans and 21 ring dips; the second would be 15 cleans and 15 dips; and the last round would be 9 cleans and 9 dips. There was no rest between sets or rounds—it was about how fast he could do the whole program. Comments indicated that people were finishing the workout in 5 to 10 minutes. Widman reasoned that with his extensive background, supreme dedication, and U.S. Marine-cut mental toughness, 5 to 10 minutes seemed reasonable. He pushed start on a stopwatch and began his first CrossFit workout.

Fifty-eight minutes later, Widman finished, "prostrate in a puddle of bodily fluids," he recalls. "It broke my ego. But this type of training was what I'd been looking for my whole life." He launched himself into it, and his passion was duly noted; from the beginning, CrossFit was heavily connected to law enforcement and the military, and Widman's leadership role with the Marines attracted CrossFit Headquarters. He was invited to help at the fledgling seminars where new coaches were being trained. He began to teach CrossFit, and it became a way of life. Widman now leads CrossFit Level 1 coaching certifications for a living.

Formerly a national-class kayaker, Kelly Starrett—my coach at the CrossFit Open qualifying event—was working on his doctorate in physical therapy when, while web surfing one night, he landed on the CrossFit site. Starrett's career as a kayaker had slammed to a halt at the same time that his interest in physical therapy was born, when one day his muscles seized up and he couldn't turn his head. This event had sparked an interest in the deeper fundamentals of human movement. He and his wife, Juliet, would eventually start a CrossFit gym in their backyard, with their landlord as its first member. CrossFit would influence Starrett's philosophy as a physical therapist to the point that he now openly criticizes the business of sports medicine with incendiary vigor. Demand for his services comes from Tour de France cyclists, world-record-holding power lifters, San Francisco ballet stars, U.S. Special Forces personnel, and Navy SEALs.

These are just some of the stories that buzz throughout the world of CrossFit—a nontraditional form of exercise and nutrition that is also called "the Sport of Fitness." Similar accounts have come from housewives, Mixed Martial Arts (MMA) fighters, former drug addicts, and many others. As a result, the sport has been given credit for turning the conventional route of fitness inside out.

My introduction to CrossFit was via yet another route, one that has been traveled by fellow runners before me. It's the path of the broken runner: the seemingly never-ending, continually frustrating cycle of injury that comes with training for and racing marathons, half-marathons, 10Ks, and other races. Some 70 percent of runners get injured every year, and some of us, with desperation in our eyes, have limped into a CrossFit gym looking for an answer. This was most certainly the case for me.

BREAKING DOWN

Late October 2010: It was a humid Sunday morning in Southern California, and I had less than 400 yards to go to finish the Rock 'n' Roll Half Marathon in Los Angeles. I was miserable, wanting relief from the leg and knee pains that had gnawed at my joints each step of the hilly 13-mile route that circuited downtown LA.

Within 200 yards of the race finish near LA Live, the 5.6-million-square-foot complex of hotels, restaurants, and high-tech stadium theaters next to the Staples Center, I was unable to muster any zip in my finishing sprint.

I crossed the line and walked out of the chute, through the typical mayhem that is the finish area of a big running race. My knees were burning with a smoldering ache; it felt like the interior cartilage was being eaten away by sulfuric acid. I sat down on the curb and rubbed my knees with no relieving effect. As the burning heated up, I wondered how I was going to fold my legs into a Honda Fit for the two-hour drive back to San Diego.

This had been more than just a race for me. The half-marathon was part of a plan I had devised to reconstitute my physical and mental fitness after suffering a series of running injuries and a painful divorce. Unhealthy, stressed out, overweight, sleepless, aging fast, and not running had sent me nine months earlier to a local goth bar to do some introspection. I had spent a couple of weeks sitting in a dark corner of the bar, brooding. The place had brushed concrete floors and a sign with the word, scripted in a Celtic font, "PUNISHMENT." One day, I heard "Song for the Dead," by Queens of the Stone Age, being pumped through the bar's elevated speakers. It was a pivotal moment.

THIS TYPE OF TRAINING WAS WHAT I'D BEEN LOOKING FOR MY WHOLE LIFE.

I concluded that the time to act was now, that brooding through a few more months at a goth bar might just further complicate things. I committed to bashing my way back into being a runner. It would be perhaps my twentieth such post-injury comeback attempt since the mid-1990s, when my injuries had gained frequency. Comebacks rarely lasted six months before another case of Achilles' tendinitis or piriformis sciatica appeared.

Part of the problem was the load. I was overweight, with a 25 percent body-fat percentage, meaning that, at 200 pounds, it was sort of like trying to run while holding four bowling balls. Coupled with a poor diet, being sidelined by injury ultimately adds pounds. So I decided to overhaul my nutrition, too. My plan was to train for a December half-marathon and to clean up my diet by starting with a five-day juice fast. Not only that, I would adopt a vegan diet.

Running had been a part of who I was for my entire adult life. In the 1990s, I was even, at times, fairly good at it. I'd clocked a 2:38 marathon, a 15:00 5K, a 32-minute 10K, a 4:06 1,500 meters, and a 2:03 800 meters, all after I started distance running in my mid-twenties. Personal records were intermixed with the classic running injuries, though: patella tendinitis, Achilles' tendon tears, iliotibial band syndrome, piriformis sciatica, plantar fasciitis, chronic hamstring tears, muscle cramps that lasted two weeks—I'd had them all.

So, in 1997, I did what many injury-frustrated runners do. I became a triathlete. The idea was to run less but to cross-train with swimming and biking. It worked, to a degree. I would ultimately complete five Ironmans and a number of shorter races. But something deeper than surface injuries began to harm my training. I just didn't feel right. I developed slight, crooked limps. Getting out of bed in the morning was accompanied by popping, cracking, and stiffness. I had lost any sort of spring in my step. What once was running now resembled more of a slog. There was nothing pleasurable about running anymore.

Nevertheless, in 2010, as I sat there in the goth bar contemplating my limited choices, and in the worst shape I'd ever been in, running was the only place that I could return to that seemed reliable to me.

I purchased an online training plan and set a goal of running a sub-1:30 half by December, nine months away. I shopped at Whole Foods and began to live on organic produce and rice and beans. I made quinoa and oatmeal. I used a juicer. My friends at work made considerable fun of me and hinted at how much they wanted to spike my lunch with an animal-food product.

I got into the vegan thing. On Saturdays, I paid visits to a vegan-only store in the University Heights neighborhood of San Diego to hang out and talk with other vegans about what it was like to be vegan. I drank green tea with rice milk. I tried to like vegan simulations of hamburger. In three months, I lost 25 pounds, although a photo of me in August of that year shows that, while I had lost weight, it wasn't in a healthy way. I had a green hue to my skin and looked like I'd just been released from the hospital.

Meanwhile, I was tractoring through 55 to 60 miles per week. This was considerably less than my peak mileage during the 1990s. In the 1990s I would run 22 miles on Sunday, 16 miles on Friday, and hard 10-milers on Tuesdays and Thursdays. On other days I would run once in the morning and once in the evening. I was running 100 miles per week. I was running the 10-mile runs at a sub-6-minute pace, and my long runs at well under 6:30 per mile. But I had resolved not to linger on the past. It didn't matter, I decided, because this was about solving a problem in the present.

And thus it was that at that October half-marathon in Los Angeles, a hilly course, I ran as hard as I could to get a disappointing 1:37. I had six weeks to sharpen up and get under 1:30 to achieve my 2010 goal. But the smoldering knees were a sign. And in the coming weeks, things would tip from temporary injuries into the domain of the possibly permanent.

BROKEN RUNNER

On November 5, 2010, two weeks after the LA half, I was in New York City to watch the NYC Marathon. I was walking to a subway station on 50th street, after visiting the expo at the convention center, when I felt a flash of pain cut through my right knee. My leg wobbled and buckled with the pain, as if momentarily all of the connective tissue holding my knee together had disappeared. It felt as if I'd stepped into a pothole. I recovered and dismissed it as a meaningless, random occurrence not worthy of my attention. But every few minutes it would happen again, and as the day wore on the intervals between the buckling lessened. By the end of the day, I could take only two regular steps before the knee would give out. And I still had my run to do that day.

I went to a Duane Reed and spent $50 on a knee brace, wraps, Advil, and ice packs. I went to my hotel room and iced my knee to a pale blue, then put on running shoes and the brace, went to the hotel gym, and climbed on a treadmill. My training called for a tempo run, 25 minutes at 170–175 heartbeats per minute. As I was warming up, my knee collapsed several times; however, I found that if I angled my foot in a certain way, the joint held. When I started running fast, I was able to go for several minutes at a time without any problems. I finished the tempo run and checked it off my list.

But despite icing three or four times per day and taking a number of days off, as the weeks passed, the limp worsened. With worried looks, coworkers asked about me as I moved carefully about the office pulling myself along using the top frames of cubicles like rails on a stairwell.

"Are you okay? You're not going to be able to do that race, are you?"

"Oh!" I'd respond, laughing off their attention. "The funny thing is that while I can't walk, I can still run. It's strange!"

Four days before the race, I intended to do a 4-mile run, but barely made it 100 yards. My right leg had all but stopped functioning. I knew the race was over. It seemed that I would need a knee surgery soon. Perhaps a knee replacement.

The program I had been using was a standard periodization plan based on the work of the late Arthur Lydiard, a New Zealand coach whose approach is now the foundation of almost all running programs used around the world. Lydiard training started with an aerobic foundation of base mileage, which lasted for 12 weeks or more, then shifted to a hill or strength-training phase, then to a speed or track-work phase and finally a race phase. My version started with low mileage, slowly built up to 50 miles per week, and was peppered with faster runs and interval workouts. Two or three times per week, I also performed a core-strength-training program of planks and exercises with a balance ball. I had used a leg-extension machine at LA Fitness to try and resurrect my right knee. I had also stretched and done sit-ups. Yet after nine months of steady, regular work, I couldn't run 100 yards in a flat parking lot.

> HER HAMSTRINGS HAD A SHAPE AND ENERGY CHARGE THAT REMINDED ME OF A DRAWN BOW. SHE LOOKED UNBREAKABLE.

I knew the Lydiard approach worked because it was how I once had trained to run 26.2 miles at an average pace of 6:04 per mile to complete a 2:38 marathon in 1991. Not to mention that just about every distance-running great from the past 50 years had used some interpretation of Lydiard's method (if not the exact method itself). Lydiard training is, without a doubt, the most successful method employed by distance runners in modern history.

But what had worked for me in the 1990s was no longer working. I wasn't mechanically capable of carrying out the program.

"Life is short. Life is hard," said Bruce Denton, a character in the novel *Once a Runner* by John L. Parker, Jr. In the story, Denton is a 5,000-meter Olympic champion who earlier in life had won the gold medal through a high-mileage work ethic that stopped for nothing, including the inevitable physiological breakdown that occurs from overtraining. "The object, according to Denton," says the narrator, "was to 'run through' the thing, just as he maintained one should attempt to 'run through' most of those other little hubcaps life rolls into your lane; everything from death in the family to cancer of the colon." Denton ultimately turns to coaching after his running causes permanent damage to his Achilles' tendon. In a later novel, *Again to Carthage*, also by Parker, the same character can no longer run at all. He exercises by riding a mountain bike.

It's a destiny that many disciplined distance runners ultimately must confront, especially those who run for many years, and particularly if they have flawed biomechanics. Things start wearing out.

I had read another book, *Born to Run*, this one nonfiction, and had found Christopher McDougall's reporting about the Tarahumara Indians' running culture interesting. McDougall makes a strong case that the modern development of the running shoe, with built-up heels and various motion-control technologies, played a big role in producing the injuries that have become so common in the lives of American runners. Nike gets the largest share of the blame.

In *Born to Run*, McDougall recounts a transformation he experienced that included paring down to a simpler running shoe (among other things, as he also worked on his form, his strength, and his diet). The notion that running shoes were the cause of my downfall was something I considered; perhaps they had led me to poor running mechanics that had destroyed my body in an unnatural way. But I didn't think that what had sprung McDougall back to life as a runner would work for me. In the spirit of the book, I had tried running in neutral and minimal shoes, and I had already been trying to repair my stride with ancillary training—a basic core-strength program—and form correction. McDougall was able to run an ultramarathon in the depths of Mexico by the book's end. I wasn't able to even start a half-marathon on the road.

I was desperate. I was ready to try anything.

I didn't know it yet, but I was primed for CrossFit.

IS THIS FOR ME?

Early in 2010, I was running on the treadmill at an LA Fitness in Mira Mesa, a section of San Diego that is home to an array of biotech and genetic research companies. I was using the machine because the rubber belt absorbed some of the shock as compared to running on roads, enabling me to run more than I normally would be able to handle. The treadmills were located both on the second level of the gym, where you could watch cable shows from TVs that hung from the ceiling, and the main floor, where people worked out with Cybex and Universal-type machines.

One day a new personal trainer appeared. She was short and built like a gymnast—muscular, with defined arms, shoulders, and legs. Her hamstrings had a shape and energy charge that reminded me of a drawn bow. She looked unbreakable. The typical trainer-client relationship at LA Fitness consisted of a uniformed staffer walking a client from machine to machine. The typical routine included a lot of breaks and a lot of chatting, even while the client was doing shoulder presses, rows, and leg extensions. Which was one reason this new trainer stood out: She didn't go near a machine. She worked out in an open, carpeted area near the front desk, away from the machines. Her client was a middle-aged man in a white T-shirt and grey trunks. His face was red, and he was breathing hard as the trainer, circling him, shouted commands, very much like a drill sergeant getting in the face of a misbehaving soldier or a wrestling coach pushing his wrestlers in a workout.

She cycled burpees with sit-ups, jump roping, and other odd things I'd never seen before. The client would run to a wall, and from a crouched position, thrust a medicine ball upward and push it into the air so that it would bounce off the wall and back to him. Whenever the client's energy began to falter or he began to back off, the trainer would lean in and put on the pressure with verbal commands. Her mission was apparent: to get him to go to the edge of his endurance and hold it there for as long as possible. Between sets of exercises, there were no breaks or intervals. She just kept hassling him. Within seven minutes, the guy was clearly whacked—hands on his knees, staggering lightly, and with a heaving chest. And that was it; it was over. She talked to him for a while, and then he spent some time stretching and slowly walked out.

After my run I went and found the trainer and asked her what it was she was doing. She gave me a copy of a newsletter, the *CrossFit Journal*, that she said came off of an Internet site called CrossFit.com.

CrossFit.com, as it turned out, was the keyhole through which I first glimpsed what appeared to be some kind of underground society of fitness addicts. Videos on the site showed men and women, tattooed and sinewy, with four-packs and eight-packs, doing handstand push-ups, jumping onto tall boxes, hoisting large amounts of weights overhead like they do in the Olympics, climbing ropes, and using gymnastics rings. And they were doing all of this not in the polished chrome world of 40,000-square-foot fitness establishments, but in garages and backyards and industrial warehouse spaces.

Months later, after my knee had fallen apart and I began to have visions of the operating table, I started to spend more time on the CrossFit.com site. The day I started really trying to figure out what it was I was looking at, I was sitting in my office in pain. Standing up and walking to the other side of the building had become a teeth-grinding experience. I took a closer look at the newsletter the trainer had given me, which had an article entitled "Foundations." One passage immediately caught my eye. It said: "Our approach is consistent with what is practiced in elite training programs associated with major university athletic teams and professional sports. CrossFit endeavors to bring state-of-the-art coaching techniques to the general public and athlete who haven't access to current technologies, research, and coaching methods."

And then, a paragraph entitled, "Is This for Me?" read as follows: "Absolutely! Your needs and the Olympic athlete's differ by degree not kind. Increased power, strength, cardiovascular and respiratory endurance, flexibility, stamina, coordination, agility, [and] balance . . . are each important to the world's best athletes and to our grandparents."

There had been a day when I would have scoffed at all of this cross-training-style fitness talk. But my knee burned, and it felt like my back was going out as well. I had just withdrawn from the December half-marathon because I couldn't run. I couldn't remember the last time I'd felt like an athlete. It may have all been bullshit, and at the time, I suspected that it was. But that was the day I knew I had nothing to lose if I at least started looking around.

The first question I needed to answer was this: What is CrossFit?

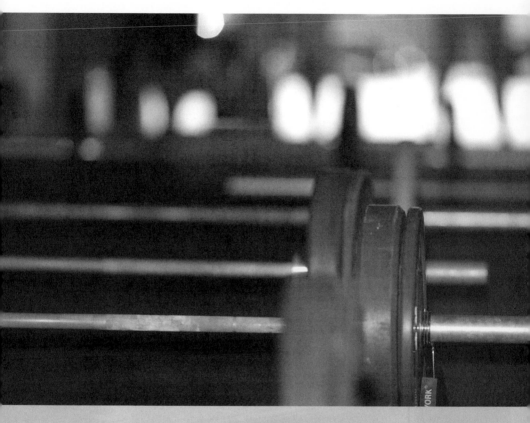

THE UNKNOWN AND
THE UNKNOWABLE

WHAT IS CROSSFIT ALL ABOUT?

2

IN THE LATE 1990S, JIM BAKER WAS A PRINCIPAL SERVING IN THE SANTA CRUZ County school system. In his down time, he worked out at what was then called the Spa Fitness Center on 41st Avenue in Capitola. One day he had a discussion about fitness with one of the gym's personal trainers, a former gymnast who had moved to Santa Cruz from Los Angeles. His name was Greg Glassman. To make a point, Glassman asked Baker if he could do a squat—with no weights, no bar, no machine. Just a basic air squat—what some might call a deep-knee bend—from a standing position. Baker didn't see much use in an air squat, since his experience of performing leg exercises at the gym was defined by the machines that were then and still are standard at modern health clubs. He was used to the kind of equipment that would guide him through routine movements such as leg extensions, leg presses, leg curls, hip abductions and adductions, calf raises, and so on.[1]

Baker was in his early fifties at the time, and a motorcycle accident had added to the general issues he already had with flexibility. This quickly became apparent, as after Baker had descended just a matter of inches downward, he could go no further. "I couldn't get back up," Baker recalls. "Coach had to pull me up by my pants."

Baker and his wife, Deb, joined Glassman's growing clientele at the gym, which included Eva Twardokens, or Eva T, as she's affectionately called, a world-class alpine skier with Olympic credentials. It became apparent to the Bakers that Glassman was an iconoclast at the Spa Fitness Center. His training methods

---

1. Information about Glassman for this chapter and all quotations by him are culled from online sources, including video archives of the *CrossFit Journal* and articles he has written. I had one meeting with Glassman, on April 5, 2012, but it was not a formal interview. Based on speeches he's given to affiliate owners, marketing through publicity is not of interest to Glassman, and while he has granted interviews to journalists in the past, Glassman's current policy seems to be that if he's going to answer questions from the media it will be within the *CrossFit Journal*. There are hours of video of Glassman discussing a range of subjects pertaining to CrossFit, and he's an excellent speaker. It is apparent that Glassman is not shackled by any traditional corporate decorum a CEO would typically use. This is evident in the quotes I've pulled. Quotes from the other sources in the book, such as Jim Baker, were obtained through interviews granted in person, over the phone, or through e-mail.

2 The Unknown and the Unknowable

differed from the common modus operandi of other personal trainers at the spa and just about anywhere else. Glassman had a history of turning a health club inside-out, bypassing, if not ignoring, the tens of thousands of dollars of gleaming chrome machines—equipped with state-of-the-art, cam-calibrated resistance delivery systems and ultra-comfortable ergonomics—and using either free weights or equipment he brought from home, such as a set of still rings.

The way Glassman had his clients use the equipment didn't go over very well with management. Instead of traditional weight training circuits that moved from machine to machine, or long, easy-to-medium efforts that took place in the cardio theater on treadmills or indoor bikes, Glassman wove together high-intensity routines that included basic gymnastics moves, classic powerlifts, Olympic-style weight lifting, running sprints, all-out rowing efforts, box-jumping, and an unorthodox use of dumbbells, which his clients seemed to furiously swing around in unusual ways. Glassman's clients jumped, heaved, and twirled in a tornadic chaos.

One day, Twardokens was slashing a barbell loaded with weights up into the air, working on Olympic lifts under Glassman's guidance, and, as happens sometimes with maximum-effort attempts on such lifts, she failed at one point and needed to dump the bar from a height above her shoulders. The bar and weights crashed to the ground, alarming the authorities. "That pretty much did it for Coach," Baker recalls. Glassman and his wife, Lauren, also a trainer employing the avant-garde style of training, were both fired.

"EVEN THEN, GREG HAD THIS VISION," BAKER REMARKS WHEN RECALLING THE STORY. "HE'D SAY, 'WE'RE GOING TO CHANGE THE WAY THE WORLD THINKS ABOUT FITNESS.'"

Baker was at work when Glassman phoned to tell him the news. It was not a new experience for Glassman—he had been kicked out of an assortment of other gyms in the Los Angeles area for much the same reason, but Southern California had an inexhaustible supply of gyms. Get kicked out of one, pack up and move to the next, a few miles down the road. Smaller than LA County by many millions, Santa Cruz offered fewer options. Baker was on the phone with Glassman, and between Baker's fingers was a new credit card he'd just received in the mail. Baker proposed to Glassman that maybe he should just get his own place. "I have this new Visa card," he told Glassman. "You could use it to buy some equipment and go out on your own."

"Even then, Greg had this vision," Baker remarks when recalling the story. "He'd say, 'We're going to change the way the world thinks about fitness.' But here he was. He and Lauren were living in a little place in Santa Cruz. They didn't even have cars, and now they didn't have jobs. I knew Greg was either a genius or a lunatic . . . or maybe both. But we decided to follow him."

Glassman bought a few dumbbells, a barbell, and a rowing machine and rented 400 square feet of space in the corner of Claudio França's Brazilian Jiu-Jitsu studio. Most of his clients followed him. Glassman set his alarm for 4 a.m. and would usually be wide-awake much earlier, in fear that he'd miss the alarm. He'd grab a quick breakfast and bike to work in the dark, and sometimes in the rain. He'd train clients from 5 a.m. into the evening. The business began to grow, and the Glassmans moved to larger spaces, eventually leasing the first CrossFit Headquarters at 2851 Research Park Drive in the eastern part of Santa Cruz– a space that had the size and look of a one-car garage. But this time, it was all theirs.

Word got around that a new gym with an extreme training method was producing extreme results. Much of the training spilled out into the six-space parking lot or took place in runs back and forth to a nearby FedEx facility. More people came. CrossFit HQ took over the adjacent space and now occupied an area that was more like the size of a two-car garage.

In 2002, Glassman started giving seminars to explain what he was doing. CrossFit began posting workouts for free on the Internet. An online magazine was started, videos were posted, and Glassman's students began opening their own CrossFit gyms. By 2005, there were 13 of these affiliates. By 2012, there would be more than 4,000. CrossFit.com gets 150,000 visitors per day.

DEFINING CROSSFIT

Just what was Glassman's vision? And what is CrossFit? Is it a paradigm-shifting fitness revolution? Yes. Is it a submission into the $25 billion fitness-club industry that does almost everything differently? Yes again. Is it a fitness approach that serves up workouts that, if performed as prescribed, may kill you? Well, yes. Is it a cyber-based web/social-networking communication portal? Undoubtedly.

And more: CrossFit is a high-intensity exercise program known to achieve stunning results in a short burst of time. It's a platform enabling a new generation of bodybuilding-like narcissists to flood the web with what might be classified as soft-core fitness erotica. It's an unusual method of combining exercise, diet, and support in such a way that it is saving lives. It's an open-source collaboration among a wide range of experts from a diaspora of sports, such as gymnastics, weight lifting, and running. It's the brainchild of a charismatic, self-taught guru with genius-like abilities in math, science, and physiology, who is, by his own admission, "pretty fucking arrogant," and it's a movement supported by a rabid, impassioned throng of followers who buy and swap T-shirts the way philatelists collect stamps. And it's a televised sport with elite super-athletes, which doesn't stop it from being an antitechnology grassroots community-builder that is serving almost as a church for some of its devotees.

The roots of Glassman's vision lie in an experience he had when he was 10 years old. Growing up in the San Fernando Valley in California—"in a family of rocket scientists that lived in a neighborhood of rocket scientists"—he sometimes received unusual assignments from his father, an engineer who worked on the weapons systems of fighter planes. One day his dad handed him a micrometer and a sack full of nails, labeled "1000 NAILS," and told him to measure each nail with the micrometer to the 1,000th of an inch and graph the frequencies of the lengths. He wanted to teach him about data collection. "I hated the old man for that one," Glassman says. It seemed a tiresome, useless task. But at the end of the drudgery, he was shocked to see that the dots on the graph took the shape shown in Figure 2.1.

It was a Gaussian curve, otherwise known as the bell curve, a normal distribution, generated from a sack of 1¾-inch nails. "It was profound," Glassman

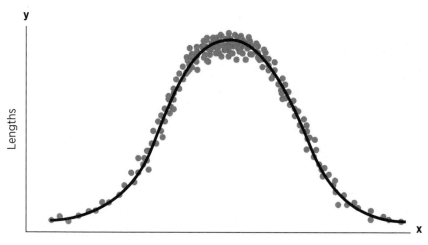

FIGURE 2.1 GRAPH OF A BELL CURVE

y

Lengths

x

Number of nails

says. "The fabric of the universe or some miracle of understanding so breathtaking in its simplicity and elegance arising out of observation and careful measurement." The experiment taught Glassman to reserve his judgments, basing them on his own observations and experiments, and to be highly dubious of the beliefs and methodologies of others if they didn't have the kind of data that could sway him.

A highly curious individual, he frequently used experimentation to solve problems. By 1971, Glassman was a determined high-school gymnast without year-round access to a gym. His specialty was the still rings—two wooden rings connected by straps to a metal frame that are used in events known for requiring tremendous amounts of upper-body strength. In the Iron Cross, for example, the athlete suspends himself in the air, arms extended out within the horizontal plane of the body, for at least two seconds. But it wasn't just sheer strength that Glassman wanted to build in the off-season; it was muscular stamina, as demanded by his sport.

GLASSMAN WANTED THAT QUEASY FEELING OF BEING ANAEROBICALLY BLOWN APART. SOMETHING THAT WOULD RAMP UP HIS CONDITIONING AND ALLOW HIM TO STICK A RINGS ROUTINE AS IF HE HAD FINISHED NOTHING MORE TAXING THAN A CARD TRICK.

A well-executed routine in gymnastics, such as a two-minute routine on the parallel bars with handstands, flips, and presses, is a graceful display of strength, power, and flexibility. But also at play are stamina and endurance. The roles that these qualities play may not be apparent to an observer, because one of the many tasks of the competitive gymnast is to hide the appearance of effort. To avoid point deductions, a gymnast must land a routine in a way that sheds no clue about the stamina that's being channeled from the engine to perform the routine. The external image may appear controlled, but the muscular recruitment and power demands of a two-minute routine on the parallel bars or rings are massive.

The teenage Glassman wanted a head start in the off-season, and without gym access, wondered what he could do on his own with weight training. His dad helped the experiment along. The '63 station wagon was backed out of the garage, which was then turned into a gym. The initial investment was a Ted Williams set of weights, $19.95 at Sears and Roebuck, and an AMF pull-up bar screwed into a doorframe. The weight set consisted of blue plastic weights filled with concrete, a barbell, and a pamphlet showing the basic exercises.

Trying out exercises like arm curls, from the Ted Williams pamphlet, left the young Glassman underwhelmed. The effort required was pitiful compared to even a minute on the parallel bars. "I needed something that would leave you sitting on your ass gasping for air, like a rings routine." He also wanted to simulate the compound movements made in gymnastics, and an exercise like the barbell curl, which isolated the bicep, didn't do the job. Glassman wanted that queasy feeling of being anaerobically blown apart. Something that would ramp up his conditioning and allow him to stick a rings routine as if he had finished nothing more taxing than a card trick.

Glassman began to create his own exercises and mix them up with body-weight gymnastics moves he could do in the garage. Holding the barbell on his shoulders, under his chin, he would squat down as far as he could, then explode upward, driving the weights toward the ceiling until his arms were locked out as in a completed press. It was essentially the combination of a front squat and a push press. "The thruster was born," he says. Ten thrusters in a row started to give him the feeling he was seeking.

With the loaded barbell, Glassman arbitrarily came up with a sequence of numbers: 21, 15, 9. In his attempt to simulate the effort of a rings routine, he would perform, as fast as he could get through it, the following workout:

21 thrusters

21 pull-ups

15 thrusters

15 pull-ups

9 thrusters

9 pull-ups

After finishing the final pull-up, a shaken Glassman vomited all over the garage floor. In an act that presaged his eventual career as a personal trainer, the young gymnast, still wearing his vomit-stained shirt, then managed to lure a neighbor buddy, a curious teammate, into the garage, where they repeated the workout. They both threw up.

Glassman has articulated that the heart of CrossFit has essentially been reverse engineered from this vomit-triggering workout he'd stumbled upon.

What Glassman said he liked about it was that it produced the same feeling you'd get after a hard gymnastics routine, or, as police officers would later tell him, it left you feeling the same way you did after a long foot chase that turned into a fight. It delivered the athlete into the raw discomfort of an anaerobic state of effort and training effect.

Research that began accumulating in the 1990s and after would support the concept of HIIT, "High Intensity Interval Training," as being a superior form of exercise than slower, longer, aerobic types of training. From HIIT training, you gain more of a fat-burning effect, spur a release of human growth hormone, decrease cellular inflammation, and are able to belt out more performance. One such demonstration on the performance effect of high-intensity spurts of interval work appeared in a 2005 study published in the *Applied Journal of Physiology* that put eight college-age subjects—all considered "recreationally active"—through two weeks of interval workouts. Six of the subjects doubled their endurance (as defined by how long they could ride on a bike until exhaustion). While the compound exercises (and combinations of exercises) change on a daily basis, workouts at CrossFit are almost universally performed in these sorts of interval or time-trial formats.

The 21-15-9 workout with thrusters and pull-ups remains today the most famous workout in the CrossFit world. Like all CrossFit benchmark workouts, it has a name: "Fran." The reason Glassman began naming workouts is that it was much easier to explain the details of a workout once and then refer to it henceforth by a name. "It takes five minutes to explain the fucker," Glassman says in a CrossFit.com video. "I wanted to explain it once and give it a name." Asked why the benchmark workouts have been given girls' names, Glassman replied, "I thought that anything that left you flat on your back looking up at the sky asking, 'What the fuck happened to me?' deserved a female's name. . . . If hurricanes that wreak havoc on a town can be given a name, so can a workout."

Fran has such a legendary status in the CrossFit world that the most universal of CrossFit T-shirts is imprinted with, "For a good time, call Fran: 21-15-9."

DEFINING FITNESS

Glassman became an all-around athlete, but with an odd combination of interests. He loved gymnastics and riding bicycles, and now he loved weight training. "Someone might be able to beat me in one of the disciplines, but I could usually crush him in the other two," he says. By age 16, Glassman had begun to coach, training track-and-field athletes in basic gymnastics skills to improve their power.

Thanks in part to living near the mecca of bodybuilding, Gold's Gym at Venice Beach, a place where the world's best bodybuilders trained (most notably Arnold Schwarzenegger), Glassman came to a key realization: Just because bodybuilders *looked* like super-athletes didn't mean they *were* super-athletes. Glassman could see that all the muscle and definition achieved through the bodybuilding routines being employed at Gold's were superficial; maybe it got them into a beefcake calendar, but it didn't translate into athletic facility.

Glassman's irreverent nature bloomed in his college years at the same time a passion for math and physics took hold of him, although he also pursued studies in literature. By the time the health-club boom began to sweep America, Glassman had seen enough to question the methods being advocated by the health clubs. He had also noticed the competition that had emerged among manufacturers of fitness machines, companies such as Nautilus, Universal, Cybex, and so on. Glassman would rapidly develop skepticism of the machines that isolated individual muscles. From his perspective, there was no comparing the effectiveness of a $15 pull-up bar that you screwed into a doorframe versus, for example, a chain-and-camshaft-driven machine designed to work the bicep that cost thousands of dollars and weighed hundreds of pounds.

Glassman had become consumed with unlocking the power he'd found in his Fran workout, and in so doing he was hearing what he found to be nonsense coming from exercise science. If exercise, fitness, and health are going to be a science, Glassman reasoned, then, first of all, don't we need to define the terms? What is "fitness"? What is "health"?

Glassman searched for concrete definitions—concrete enough that they would make sense to an engineer or a physicist. He combed through the definitions provided by the various exercise-science organizations, such as the American College of Sports Medicine, but everything seemed too broad and fuzzy (such as health being defined as "the absence of disease"). It was as if the people who were coming up with the definitions were trying to please everyone who had something to gain from what the definition was—or as if they'd invited a yoga practitioner, a runner, a weight lifter, an aerobics instructor, and a step-class enthusiast into a conference room and wouldn't let anyone leave the room until they'd come up with a definition that everyone could live with.

Glassman reasoned that without a proper definition, a personal trainer had no clear objective to strive for, and hence proper measurement couldn't take place. How do you know what you're achieving or not achieving if you haven't arrived at a clear definition? When I met Glassman, he was talking to a group of CrossFit HQ associates at a baseball game outing, recounting a recent explanation he'd given to outsiders of why you need a definition of fitness. He said, "Let's say we all decide we want to know how many crickets there are in a field. First thing, we need to come to an agreement on what a cricket is. If you're out there counting what you think are crickets and I'm out there counting what I think are crickets, but because we haven't agreed on what a cricket is we're counting all sorts of bugs, we're nowhere. The first thing we have to do is decide what a fucking cricket is." The ideas, experiments, and conclusions that coaches and trainers were taking for granted had no real basis. Without definitions, Glassman insisted, you didn't have measurement, and without either, you weren't doing science.

A definition was needed, so Glassman began developing his own. He wanted a general definition of fitness that cut to the bone in a scientific way.

GPP: THE BROAD VIEW OF FITNESS

As Glassman considered the flawed definitions of fitness he had come across, he determined, in his own definition, to argue against the idea that the height of fitness was winning the Tour de France or the Hawaii Ironman, bench-pressing 700 pounds, or becoming Mr. Olympia. Glassman was dubious when *Outside* magazine, in 1997, declared six-time Ironman champion Mark Allen as the fittest man alive. For Glassman, there was no denying Allen's greatness as an athlete, but then, what about a champion decathlete? Or world champions from swimming, weight lifting, gymnastics, or rowing? In evaluating fitness, which qualities were to count—strength and coordination, speed and power, or stamina and endurance? How should these be weighed?

Glassman concluded that specializing at a sport was at odds with the mission of his job as a personal trainer: to help others pursue a high degree of general fitness. A pure health and fitness program should prepare a client for a wide range of physical applications. He wanted a CrossFit athlete to hit a variety of targets equally well, as opposed to hitting one or two targets and leaving the others to rot. So, first he borrowed a list of skills from the makers of the Dynamax® medicine ball that he felt did a good job of covering all the bases:

Endurance

Stamina

Strength

Flexibility

Coordination

Balance

Agility

Accuracy

Power

Speed

"You are as fit as you are competent in each of these ten skills," Glassman wrote in the *CrossFit Journal* in 2002. "A regimen develops fitness to the extent that it improves each of these 10." Glassman also noted that endurance, stamina, strength, and flexibility are improved through training; coordination, balance, agility, and accuracy were improved by practice; and speed and power came through a combination of training and practice.

For this state of readiness, he coined a term: General Physical Preparedness, or GPP. Glassman argues that knowing what your GPP is will allow you to spot weaknesses so that you can focus your training, practice, and improve.

POWER: THE CURRENCY OF FITNESS

To define and measure the status of these 10 capacities in an athlete, Glassman believes that there is only one valid metric, the same metric that would be used to evaluate a racecar: power. Power, as an engineer would define it, is force times distance divided by time. For example, if you have a sandbag that weighs 50 pounds (that is, it is being pulled toward the earth with a force of 50 pounds), and you lift it 1 foot in 1 second, your power output is 50 foot-pounds per second. In the metric system, the unit of measure is watts.

By measuring power output on different occasions set apart by training, Glassman concluded, you can measure improvement. If I measure my power output when lifting the 50-pound sandbag before and after training for a month, I can compute how much more power I am now able to produce, and hence, how much more fit I am. This is how Glassman ideally likes to see a CrossFit workout measured, explained, and studied, and he likes to use movements that can work with the power model cleanly and easily. When a bunch of people keep track of all weights, times, and distances in a given workout, they can rank themselves according to power output, thus gaining an understanding of how their engines compare in performance.

For Glassman, the power being produced during exercise is the very thing we should be talking about when we talk about workout or training intensity.

WHEN YOU CAN MEASURE SOMETHING, GLASSMAN THUS NOTICED, YOU ARE NOT ONLY DOING SCIENCE— YOU CAN TURN ANY MEASURABLE ACTIVITY INTO A COMPETITION.

Glassman's models in fact suggest that power and intensity are the same thing. He does not use corollaries of intensity, such as heart rate. Heart rate, he says, is a by-product of intensity, not intensity itself. Nor does he pay attention to body-fat percentages or blood pressure. The accurate measurement of power would become the currency of his entire training program. Power-output data could be measured and plotted on a graph, just like the lengths of a bag's worth of nails.

When you can measure something, Glassman thus noticed, you are not only doing science—you can turn any measurable activity into a competition. Get together a group of people, line them up with a CrossFit workout that can be measured in foot-pounds per minute or watts, get out your stopwatch, and at the end of the workout, when everyone is done, you'll have a first-place finisher, a second-place finisher, and so on. You've turned fitness into a sport. This had never before been done with traditional gym workouts. It was completely new.

Being able to measure gains in performance in a meaningful way was an extension of where Glassman was heading with his definition of fitness. Glassman found that he could take an athlete, measure the distance that he or she moved weights and/or the body in each repetition, clock the workout, and get a number that could be recorded in a log. He could then have the same athlete come back to the same workout four weeks later, clock it again, and see if there was any improvement (and if so, how much). The athlete might shave 30 seconds off of his time for the workout, or lift more weight, or both. Glassman could plug the new numbers into the power-output formula (power = [force × distance] ÷ time), log them onto the graph, and watch power output improve.

Glassman was moving in on his definition of fitness, one that may not have pleased exercise scientists at that time but pleased his engineering and math friends immensely. He took it to them, and they said, "Yes, that's it. Of course." The power-output view of exercise allowed him to observe fitness through a lens that brought it into perfect focus–the focus of Newtonian mechanics. He was now ready to declare a new definition of fitness, and his precise definition was this: "work capacity measured over broad time and modal domains."

Glassman loved that his definition allowed him to construct a graph. It's the same type of graph that every high-schooler knows from algebra, with X and Y axes at right angles. And with time progressing along the X-axis from left to right, and power output then plotted vertically from low to high over time, every CrossFit enthusiast could have a record of his or her fitness improvement.

The power-output model could be applied to anything from running to a pull-up to weight lifting to a push-up, to how far you can throw a softball, or even to a combination of all of those things in a single workout. A trainer could come up with events and combinations of movements that would take anywhere from a second or two to twenty minutes or more, collect the data from those workouts, and plot the results on the graph. Just as Glassman found when he was a child measuring nails, a pattern would begin to emerge.

For example, an athlete could plot personal records for exercises that ranged from a few seconds but demanded a large amount of power within those seconds (e.g., a deadlift or a squat) to a 5,000-meter time trial on a rowing machine that would spread the power output over 20 minutes or so. Since most CrossFit exercises are chosen so that the movements can be recorded in terms of power output and time, just about every workout you do in a CrossFit box could be turned into a data point for the graph. A curve develops, and as Coach Glassman would explain to you, the area under the curve is the visual representation of your current state of fitness. Deviations in the curve might also expose areas where you're especially strong or especially weak (see Figure 2.2).

Furthermore, the more widely varied the skills and drills plucked from across Glassman's list—endurance, stamina, strength, flexibility, power, speed, coordination, agility, balance, accuracy—the more complete the picture of the individual athlete's fitness. Fitness could be measured not in terms of how capable a person was in the margins—how fast he could run a marathon or how much weight she could bench-press, but in terms of how good the individual was at all of these qualities combined. The better someone was at all of the skills and drills, the better he could perform at just about any activity or sport thrown at him—that is, the higher his General Physical Preparedness, or GPP.

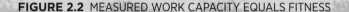

FIGURE 2.2 MEASURED WORK CAPACITY EQUALS FITNESS

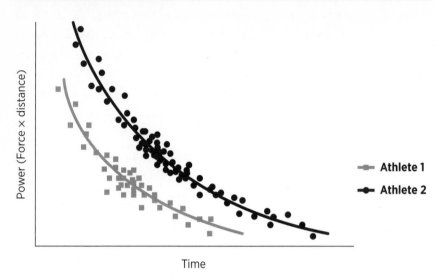

A power output graph for two athletes, per Glassman's definition of fitness. Workout results are plotted on the graph in terms of power (distance that weight is moved) and time. The resulting curve, Glassman maintains, is a graphical representation of an athlete's current fitness.

To get a quality portrait of an athlete's overall fitness—to get the measurements needed to track progress toward GPP and compare athletes in terms of it—Glassman required that the subject be tested across both broad time domains (from the couple of seconds it takes to do a one-rep max deadlift to a 5K or 10K run) and broad modal domains (the more of the 10 skills and drills you test the athlete for, the more complete the picture). This, he said, allowed the trainer and athlete to see how the athlete performed over the complete range of metabolic capacities, or the three metabolic engines that get tapped in a workout: phosphagen, glycolytic, and oxidative. Phosphagen refers to short-duration, high-power exercise that takes less than 10 seconds to complete, like a max deadlift. Glycolytic refers to exercise of moderate duration and moderate power, such as a 500-meter time trial on the rower. And oxidative means long-duration tests, such as a 10K run. A proper graph showing an athlete's fitness includes data from workouts that channel all of these energy systems.

An athlete training at a CrossFit affiliate, or following the workouts of the day (WODs) online, will be able to graph this fitness portrait if he or she keeps a journal and records numbers from workouts.

Along with power, there are three key components of Glassman's explanation of CrossFit that help to explain the method behind the seeming madness. First is the idea of preparing for the unknown; second is that routine is to be shunned in favor of a vibrant variety of workouts; third is the meaning of the third axis of the graph in its 3D version.

"The Unknown and the Unknowable"

Athletic specialists train for a specific event—for example, Lance Armstrong trained for the Tour de France, and pretty much only the Tour de France. Glassman believes that true fitness is distinctly different from this kind of specialist fitness. Fitness, he said, should be a measure of how well a person can respond to an unforeseen event, what he calls "the unknown and the unknowable."

In seminar talks, he asks his audience to consider the situation of a fireman arriving on the scene of a burning skyscraper. He doesn't know what's slated for the night's event. His preparation for that moment has to be general, as he must be ready for many possible scenarios that might emerge. Will he have to carry 200 pounds on his back up a ladder in 40 seconds? Will he have to run and jump? Scale a wall and sprint through burning rooms? All of the above? The fireman doesn't have the luxury of knowing what's going to be asked of him when the alarm goes off and the game is on. He doesn't have the luxury of training for nine months for the world-championship 1,500-meter run. It's the same with a soldier or a cop. This is what Glassman has in mind when he thinks of fitness: the broadest scope of athletic ability that one might need to tap into when it's a matter of life and death.

And this, essentially, is the format of the CrossFit Games. Athletes don't know what the events are going to be until the week of the competition. They have to prepare for the Games as broadly as possible.

Routine Is the Enemy

"Constantly varying" are key words embedded in the definition of CrossFit, and they're key to Glassman's vision. CrossFit programming is such that what the athlete does today is different from what she did yesterday, or what she will do tomorrow. CrossFitters find out what the workout will be, at best, the day before—and at some gyms they don't know until they've walked into the box. The WOD is a constant surprise, a way to shock the body so that the body never falls into a rut. Perhaps Glassman saw personal trainers during all his years at

Gold's Gyms putting clients through the same routine, day after day and year after year. Or maybe he saw that the athletes were doing the same things over and over again, and were mystified about why they were not progressing. At CrossFit, you'll hear this phrase a lot: "Routine is the Enemy." It's part of the "Hopper Model" aspect of CrossFit that Glassman talks about: Put the skills and drills in a hopper and pull out a few pieces at random, and there's your workout—3, 2, 1, go. This is a way to prepare a firefighter or soldier for "the unknown and the unknowable."

Lon Kilgore, an exercise physiologist who has studied CrossFit, feels that this is an aspect of CrossFit that can be problematic, because if workouts are chosen randomly an athlete loses out on the value that can be obtained through targeted programming, attacking specific goals with specific workouts. "Even though I heartily agree with the goal stated for the model," he says, "if I am choosing something at random, while I may be picking the right thing, I am as likely to choose an exercise or work scheme that doesn't contribute to fitness gain."

> **THE BETTER SOMEONE WAS AT ALL OF THE SKILLS AND DRILLS, THE BETTER HE COULD PERFORM AT JUST ABOUT ANY ACTIVITY OR SPORT THROWN AT HIM.**

Kilgore believes that leaving less to chance will allow a CrossFit coach to spur the trainee on to more progress, even if it removes the element of suspense that many CrossFitters find exciting. "If we intelligently choose the exercise and work schemes and program them, we will likely be better able to drive fitness gain," he noted. "I strongly believe programming works in the context of CrossFit; however, yes, it might take a little of the fun out. Not knowing what WOD awaits at the gym is like opening presents at Christmas; you look forward to finding out what's inside the box."

The Graph's Third Axis

Glassman added a third axis to the graph to produce a 3D model that further illuminates an athlete's health. This third axis measures time over a period of years. As the athlete gets older and accumulates portraits of her fitness at different ages, the graph begins to look like a drape being pulled away from a corner. The 3D area under the drape, Glassman says, is how he defines health. The athlete gets snapshots of her capacity to do all types of work, and she can see how her work capacity looks now as compared to 1 year ago, 5 years ago, or 20 years ago.

But although the third axis involves time, time—or at least longevity—is not the emphasis. In Glassman's definition of health and fitness, work capacity is the emphasis. In lectures, he warns against fixating on how long you live, or how long you avoid disease, and puts the priority instead on how well you live with the time you're given. Work capacity in your old age, Glassman says, translates into being able to live independently, being able to get up and down stairs, and being able to enjoy life. Having a great cholesterol level or blood pressure, or managing to avoid cancer, doesn't mean you have that kind of quality of life. Nor does it offer any guarantee that you will not be incapacitated by the loss of functionality, or have to be confined to a hospital bed.

The final decade of his grandmother's life had a powerful effect on Glassman's thinking. Although she was alive for those ten years, "she didn't know where she was; she didn't know who she was." She was bedridden. Glassman says that his ultimate nightmare would be that modern medicine could manage to keep him technically alive until the age of 135. He'd trade those extra years for a higher level of functional capacity for the upper register of years within a normal lifetime.

Fitness, he says, is about staying out of a nursing home and "being fed green Jello and watching Oprah all day." He says, "You want to be 90 years old, able to please your lover and beat the shit out of the punk who tries to rob you at the ATM."

SHOW, DON'T TELL

To the question of "What is CrossFit?" Glassman says that there's no simple answer. One reply he has been fond of giving is to invite the inquirer to the gym and put him through a "met-con"—that is, a metabolic-conditioning workout—that channels the same brand of anaerobic, high-intensity training that Fran is infused with. With the curious investigator flattened on his back and heaving for air, Glassman would lean over and say, "That's CrossFit."

But the language of CrossFit is changing on a daily basis, with dialects and shadings that vary from region to region, box to box. Glassman knows this. CrossFit is dynamic, and as it changes, definitions will change. Glassman says that one of the benefits of the CrossFit Games is that they may shed light on a tribe of CrossFitters somewhere that is pushing the envelope and making breakthroughs. If a small box from a small town ends up sending an inordinate number of CrossFitters to the Games, who all score exceptionally well, everyone is going to want to take a look at what they're doing.

The best way to know what CrossFit is, I found out for myself, is to join a box. I joined one with an image of what CrossFit must be firmly fixed in my mind.

I had no idea.

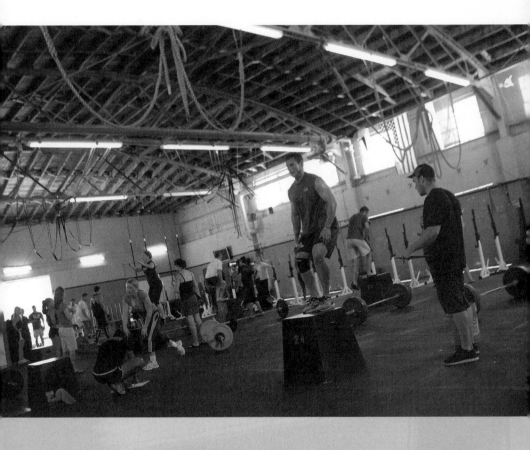

INSIDE THE BOX

THE WORLD WITHIN A CROSSFIT AFFILIATE

3

WITH AT LEAST 10 CROSSFIT AFFILIATES IN THE AREA, SAN DIEGO IS CROSSFIT-
rich. Within reach of where I lived, on 30th and Thorn in the neighborhood of
North Park—a frothy brew of hipsters, tattoo parlors, bars featuring cask beer,
vegan cafes, and fixed-gear bicycles transporting hipsters between said bars, cafes,
and tattoo parlors—I could easily drive to four CrossFit boxes. I was poised to go
check out a couple of them when I noticed that a box called CrossFit Elysium was
moving to a location very near my apartment. It would be at 30th and Adams,
a place I could get to within minutes on my one-speed Felt.

One doesn't need to join an affiliate to do CrossFit. CrossFit.com is set up to
guide someone who might be working out in a barn in the middle of the Dakota
badlands or in Bravo company of an infantry unit deployed into the field in
Afghanistan. Since February 10, 2001, a WOD has been posted every day on the
main site, and video demonstrations of the exercises are archived on a single page
of links. This is all free. Articles on how to build a home gym and follow the program online are also available. For $25 a year, you have access to the inexhaust-
ible cache of the *CrossFit Journal*, an electronic magazine brewing with a decade's
worth of articles, videos, and radio shows. And you're encouraged to post your
workout times and efforts to the forum.

GOING IT ALONE

I tried the independent route first. I was following a CrossFit endurance program designed especially for runners, attempting to execute the program at the
LA Fitness center where I was then a member. It was very "globo": a two-level
super-gym with rows of Cybex machines, free weights, dozens of cardio machines,
a basketball court, and a large room for the many classes that ran throughout the
day and night.

The first challenge in using a modern fitness center for CrossFit is simply
logistical. Say your workout of the day is supposed to be 4 rounds of 500 meters
on the rowing machine, 10 deadlifts with 125 pounds, and then 5 pull-ups. In
my case, I had to use a free-weight rack area for the deadlifts, a rowing machine
that was maybe 25 yards away, and the pull-up bar, which was near the rowing
machines. But in the area with the racks, I was in danger of tripping over the legs

of the person doing bench presses right behind me. When I left a rowing machine, more often than not I lost it to the next person waiting in line, which meant I'd have to take my chances when it was time for my next 500-meter round. It was the same with the pull-up bars. I'd jog or run to whatever area I had to use next, hoping that the equipment or space I needed wasn't already taken.

Standing and waiting for a barbell or pull-up bar means a dramatic drop in the intensity of the workout. One of the keys to building power is to keep the overall time that you're using to complete the WOD low. The obstacle-course element that came with doing the workouts in a large commercial gym made doing CrossFit sort of like trying to speed-shop at a Home Depot on a Saturday afternoon. Since I didn't have the space for a home gym at the cottage where I lived, it was my only option, but I wanted to find a better one.

Another problem, I discovered, emanated from the fact that CrossFit and traditional workouts are just two very different styles of fitness training. When people are trying to do both within the same space at the same time, collisions are inevitable. Traditional fitness training is circuit-style. People move through a predetermined pattern of exercises, going from machine to machine in a fairly quiet and orderly manner. I was first introduced to circuit-style training in 1979, when I played football in

THE FIRST CHALLENGE IN USING A MODERN FITNESS CENTER FOR CROSSFIT IS SIMPLY LOGISTICAL.

high school. My coaches installed a program based on what University of Iowa football players were doing at the time—a one set per exercise rotation through the weight room, three workouts per week, one half-hour per workout. No rest between exercises except the time it took to move from exercise to exercise. I'm not sure how effective this system was in producing good football players, but it did do one thing: It moved 60 football players through a weight training program at a considerably faster clip than the Venice Beach–style bodybuilding approach that had been in its place before. There were many sets of bench presses with huge amounts of time elapsing between each set, and everyone was in awe of the athlete with a 300-pound bench-press ability.

At LA Fitness, you can watch people doing a wide assortment of things. People wander from machine to machine, some clearly making things up as they go along. It usually works like this: You see the machines you like, grab one, do a couple of sets, then look for another machine you want to do, grab it, and so on, and a half-hour later or so you go do some cardio. Read the paper while on a Lifecycle. Or stretch. Or leave. This was how I was using LA Fitness for about three years before I started on the CrossFit path. Unsurprisingly, with my disorganized, haphazard approach, I wasn't seeing many results.

So you have people milling about from machine to machine, and here you go in with your little CrossFit battle plan requiring three or four different pieces of equipment and/or spaces. Instead of a half-hour or more, your workout would only take 12 furious minutes, if you could get the equipment and space you needed when you needed them—but no one else knows that, and why should they yield to you, anyway? So controlling access is a big problem, big enough to almost preclude doing these workouts in a busy traditional gym.

But there's another reason for the clash as well, one that is perhaps even more jarring: the aggressive nature of CrossFit is not compatible with the orderly flow that typically takes place in a commercial gym. If the two styles were different types of music, CrossFit would be the thrash death metal song next to the commercial gym's pop song. It's Napalm Death compared with Duran Duran. The harried CrossFitter thrashing his or her way through a workout designed for maximum heart rate is going against the easy-ramble grain of the others in the gym.

And then, too, if the CrossFitter is doing kettle-bell swings with a 50-pound dumbbell, and it looks like the dumbbell is going to be flung into the air, go right through the Plexiglas wall, and crash into a racquetball court, normal people tend to worry. I got many looks of concern (or maybe it was disdain) from fellow LA Fitness members. I always thought my antics would soon be stopped by a personal trainer wearing a polo shirt emblazoned with the corporate logo, who would come and tell me I was endangering others. In fact, maybe I was, but surprisingly enough, the warning never came.

Still, given the short duration of most WOD workouts, in order for them to be effective they must be high in intensity, which means they also have to be highly uncomfortable. When you are surrounded by people who are not on that same trajectory, and you know you are probably annoying them, it's hard to effectively push into the red zone. At least that's how it was for me. Sometimes I got there; sometimes I didn't. But when I finished a CrossFit workout at LA Fitness, I usually walked out feeling guilty for not having pushed as hard as I could have.

The final reason it was difficult to mesh CrossFit with a regular gym was this: CrossFit almost exclusively assigns you to do compound movements that tax the whole body—movements like squats, deadlifts, snatches, box jumps, pull-ups, and rowing. Each of the movements is technically difficult to do, and almost all of them are tricky to learn. You can watch an online video and then try to replicate the moves in the gym, but this is a precarious and possibly dangerous way to go about it. I had no one to tell me whether I was performing the movements correctly or to help me make the adjustments I needed in order to perform them safely. Injury seemed imminent.

So when CrossFit Elysium came up on the radar, and I saw that it was within biking distance on a one-gear bike, I decided to join.

CROSSFIT ELYSIUM

Elysium is that "place at the ends of the earth to which certain favored heroes were conveyed by the gods after death," according to *The New Oxford American Dictionary*. Or, "a place or state of perfect happiness." In other words, in Greek mythology, this was where certain lucky mortals were admitted for their retirement after successfully completing their heroic deeds. If you are picturing fields of flowers, shaded streams, and peaceful realms, however, think again.

CrossFit Elysium was set up in a retail/warehouse space, right next door to a dealer specializing in classic cars. A half-block south, another used-car dealership specialized in used police cars—the black and white now faded and the sirens and lights long since removed. A half-block north was a tattoo and piercing shop; across the street, another tattoo and piercing shop; on the next block, yet another tattoo and piercing shop. Most importantly, a few blocks south of Elysium was the Toronado, the unofficial bar of Elysium folk. A low-key place with picnic tables and a small beer garden, the Toronado had a close and fond relationship with the heroes of Elysium.

I'd dabbled a bit in CrossFit by the time I decided to join Elysium on July 1, 2011, but I really didn't know much about it. The one thing I did know was that Elysium would be its own world—that because of the way the overall CrossFit business model operates, the owners were free to create the character of the gym. CrossFit is not a franchise system like Starbucks or Gold's Gym, where everything is standardized in policies handed down from above, but rather, a web of affiliates. This has huge implications for the way CrossFit gyms operate.

Affiliation is a straightforward process. To apply, you need only successfully complete the two-day Level 1 coaching certification seminar and fill out an application, which includes an essay. Once you're accepted, you pay a $3,000 per year fee. From there on, the directive is fairly broad: According to the CrossFit.com website, "CrossFit is not a franchise and never will be. Our affiliates constitute a confederation of legitimate fitness practitioners united around constantly varied, intense, functional exercise and pooling reliable resources under the CrossFit name." With such a liberal amount of wiggle room, affiliates can vary widely in terms of personality, equipment, coaching quality, average class size, and emphasis. Costs also vary.

With this in mind, I walked through the glass door at Elysium for the first time, wondering what this particular world would be like. The first space I came to was wide open, with a low ceiling, pillars, and, immediately to the left, a reception desk built with planks of plywood. There was a table behind the desk with a coffee pot and a plastic tub of protein powder. Sitting at the desk working at a computer was a man with a black mop of curly hair, which sprouted from beneath a red cap. He didn't really look up as I approached the desk, only shooting me a quick glance from the corner of his eyes. I later learned this was Paul Estrada, the co-owner of the gym and the primary coach.

"Hi," Estrada said.

"Hi."

Pause.

I continued. "So . . . well, I'd like to join."

"O.K."

Pause.

Estrada's eyes darted to the computer screen and back.

"Uh, so how does that work?" I asked.

Finally looking up, Estrada quickly explained in as few words as possible that I could start attending the fundamentals classes next week.

Fundamentals, or "on-ramp" programs, as some CrossFit gyms call them, vary from affiliate to affiliate. At Elysium, you attend these scheduled classes for about a month to learn the basic movements without weights and with little or no intensity. You get a feel for the flow of the workouts, and you learn the meaning of terms like "push press" and "box jump." You learn how to perform squats—not with tons of weight on your shoulders, but with a section of nearly weightless PVC pipe, or with no equipment at all. You also get trained in how to take care of the equipment you use. Personal trainers at a Gold's Gym and other large fitness centers may do the work of loading or unloading weights and in general cleaning up after you. Not so at CrossFit gyms. During the on-ramp program, any such expectations of the coach serving you in this way give way to CrossFit's tough-love approach. If you use a barbell and two 25-pound bumper plates, then you put back the barbell and the bumper plates when you're finished.

Another sign of the tough-love approach that you see for the first time in these classes is the penalty board. Certain violations earn you burpees. Knocking into another CrossFitter with the equipment you're using, for example, comes with a serious penalty at Elysium, in the form of 200 burpees. Being a minute late costs you a few, but every additional minute you're late for the workout increases the burpee count like compound interest.

Fundamentals classes can deflate some of the fear and uncertainty new-comers commonly have. A CrossFit gym, a good one anyway, ensures that new gym members are treated the same as the hotshot who can rip through 50 pull-ups at a clap—in fact, that hotshot is often the first to congratulate you when you get your first push-up or pull-up or reach some other breakthrough goal. This holds true for the newcomer who is out of shape as well as for the newcomer who has been doing other sports but is discovering CrossFit for the first time.

I felt like I already knew enough about CrossFit to skip fundamentals, and I didn't want to wait until the next week to get started. I wanted to start that day, so I asked if I could skip the preliminary program. Estrada looked dubious but agreed, cautioning that if they saw me struggling in the workouts, they would bump me back and make me take the fundamentals.

I handed him my credit card and he scanned it. He gave me a thin welcome handout, stapled together at the corner, with the CrossFit Elysium logo on the front page. That was it. I was a member.

"There's a workout tonight," he said. "And then there's one on Sunday. And we're open on Monday." Then he looked back at his computer.

Monday was July 4.

"I'll be in tonight," I said.

BIRTH OF A BOX

Elysium had been in business for about a year and a half before moving to my neighborhood in June 2011. Estrada and co-owner Leon Chang had been training partners in Chang's backyard gym when both were new converts to the CrossFit style of training. Estrada had been a personal trainer at a 24-Hour Fitness.

Estrada's conversion to CrossFit came the first time he performed Fran at the 24-Hour Fitness facility and collapsed onto the floor from the effort.

"I couldn't move for a half-hour," he told me. "Then I finally was able to sit up. It took another 20 minutes before I could walk. I thought I knew how to train before that point. I thought I knew how to train, how to train people, and I felt I trained hard. Everything changed."

Chang's entry into CrossFit came about when his wife hired one of their friends as a personal trainer. "He was a former Marine and had been a fitness instructor for years," Chang told me. "He had just learned of CrossFit a few months before and was a CrossFit certified trainer. As we were all friends, he let me jump in on a few training sessions."

"Those first sessions just killed me," Chang says. "I was a former swimmer and soccer player and considered myself pretty athletic, so it was humbling to get crushed by some simple body-weight movements and a little bit of weight." Chang's progress was swift: He went from 175 pounds to 145 pounds, his "fighting weight," and was hooked.

Chang started training with Estrada and began building a backyard gym. He bought a squat rack, a barbell, and bumper plates and had a pull-up bar installed. "We were doing workouts most days of the week and usually could find a way to do almost every movement with the limited equipment and space we had," Chang says. He then attended a Level 1 CrossFit seminar. "Paul started bringing some of his personal clients over to train at my house," he recalls. "At our busiest we would have five people or so all working out in the garage or on the sidewalk while the neighbors would gather and watch." By late 2009, Estrada and Chang had decided to open up a CrossFit gym.

Estrada borrowed money from his family so that he could make that initial investment with Chang. They used the equipment from Chang's home gym and purchased more to supplement it. Clients came with them, and, to Estrada's relief, word began to get around. Membership in the gym slowly grew. According to Chang, after one year, CrossFit Elysium had 50 members. By then they had outgrown the space in more ways than one.

For one thing, CrossFit is a noisy neighbor. Unlike commercial gyms, CrossFit gyms are places where people expect weights to be dropped. Bumper plates—iron plates encased in foam—are used so that dropped weights won't break, but they are still noisy. And dropping weights is not only routine in CrossFit, especially when doing, for example, Olympic training lifts and peak-weight deadlifts, but arguably even necessary, as it helps athletes who are pushing their limits to maintain safety. With a heavy deadlift, it would be dangerous to lower the weight slowly to the ground after a personal-record lift. The lower back muscles could be injured. Besides, putting that kind of weight down slowly is almost impossible to do. CrossFitters also typically drop weights when they "fail" at a lift—when you are trying to do a heavy overhead squat with the weight extended directly overhead, arms locked out, at peak loads, you can lose your balance. When that happens, the thing to do is to safely bail on the lift—let the weights crash to the ground while you stand several feet away, uncrushed.

Admittedly, crashing weights aren't the only source of the noise. Shouts and grunts typically accompany the crashes. Then there's the various types of metal being played during the met-con (heavy metal, black metal, speed metal, death metal, doom metal—CrossFit gyms seem to have a taste for the apocalypse). And all of this noise sends all kinds of vibrations through a building. This is one reason many CrossFit affiliates are located in industrial areas, well away from sleepy residential neighborhoods. They're more likely to be found next to lumber mills, recycling centers, and demolition companies. If you have a class of 10 or more CrossFitters all dropping weights from overhead at the same time, which can happen in the early moments of a met-con, it sounds like a head-on car crash. This did not go unnoticed by the businesses next to the first CrossFit Elysium.

> "THOSE FIRST SESSIONS JUST KILLED ME," CHANG SAYS. "I WAS A FORMER SWIMMER AND SOCCER PLAYER AND CONSIDERED MYSELF PRETTY ATHLETIC, SO IT WAS HUMBLING TO GET CRUSHED BY SOME SIMPLE BODY-WEIGHT MOVEMENTS AND A LITTLE BIT OF WEIGHT."

The new space on 30th Street was an oblong warehouse, 4,200 square feet of all-concrete construction with a 25-foot ceiling. The high ceiling would facilitate rope climbs and the installation of gymnastics rings. Pull-up bars of ascending heights were screwed into the building's infrastructure along the south wall, and black rubber matting was laid in, along with lifting platforms embedded near the squat racks—3-by-3-foot squares of polished wood where Olympic lifts could be performed for maximum stability. Two ropes hung from the ceiling, one green and thick, the other thinner and in the traditional sand color. Along the east wall were stacks of bumper plates, from 45-pounders to 10-pounders, all the same circumference as traditional Olympic weights but with the protective foam. In the corner were the barbells, 45-pound bars for the men and 35-pound bars for women.

Whiteboards occupied most of the north wall (see Figure 3.1). One would hold a description of the day's workout, along with the names of everyone who worked out that day and their scores. Scores usually included two elements: how much the individual lifted during the strength part of the class (for example, "Deadlift 3 × 3, 250, 260, 270," meaning 3 sets of 3 reps with the corresponding weights), and how well the individual fared on the day's met-con. The score notes whether the individual did the workout as prescribed (RX) or scaled the workout in order to make it more doable—for example, by using a lighter weight or an easier technique (Mod, which stands for Modified).

At the end of the day, the whiteboard shows the performance of everyone who completed the day's workouts. Members of the last class of the night can see where they stand against everyone else who worked out that day, in particular any rivals who might have shown up at earlier classes.

A different whiteboard tracks personal records (PRs). Each time you seal a PR, you mark it on that board. In your first months in CrossFit, if you show up three or more times per week and truly make an effort, the PR faucet will be turned on all the way; you'll be improving in everything. It's intoxicating to see new PRs on the board every week. Every month or so, these PRs were collected by the coaches and transferred to a huge record board in the front of the gym. This board listed every CrossFit test and every standard CrossFit workout and type of lift as well as all the working PRs of the gym members.

FIGURE 3.1 TYPICAL CROSSFIT WHITEBOARDS

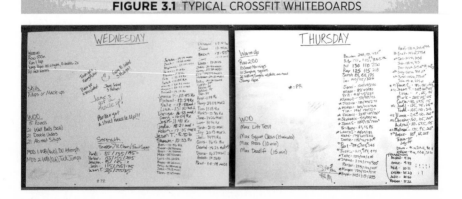

FIRST WORKOUTS

CrossFit boxes work to make newcomers feel welcome, introducing them slowly to new concepts and showing them the basics via the fundamentals program. But inevitably, in order to get results, they're going to have to enter "the pain cave," as Estrada calls it.

My first workout at Elysium consisted of the following:

WARM-UP
CF x 1

(CrossFit warm-up = 10 push-ups, 10 pull-ups, 10 back extensions, and 10 air squats)

STRENGTH
Overhead squats, 3 x 3 reps
(nightmarish for old broken former runners like me
who have no shoulder or hip mobility, core strength, or balance)

MET-CON
3 clean and jerks, 115/75 lb.
4 thrusters, 115/75 lb.
AMRAP 3 min., rest 1 min.
4 rounds total. Score is total reps.
(Note: AMRAP stands for "As Many Rounds As Possible"–
this is a common CrossFit workout format that indicates to the athlete that you're
supposed to cram in as much work as absolutely possible in the given time frame.)

Both Chang and coach Stacie Beal were in charge of the workout that day. Estrada had alerted them that I, a newbie, was going to be at the workout. When I walked in, they both greeted me warmly. One of the box members, Ben Flores, came up to me with a smile and introduced himself. So did several others. But I noticed no one was smiling when we started in on the strength workout and I attempted my first overhead squat (OHS).

Across the three sets, you're supposed to go up in weight. I started with a 45-pound bar and two 5-pound plates, for a total of 55 pounds. I got the weight overhead, but when it came time to drop into the squat I could only go a few inches. Beal gently suggested that I use the 35-pound bar with no weights—the girl bar. I took the suggestion, but my right knee had a different plan from my left knee. I looked crooked enough that Beal, again with a gentle tone, and as much positive, affirmative energy as anyone could have mustered, suggested I use a PVC pipe instead of the bar. So we started there.

Both Beal and Chang talked me through the specifics of how to do an OHS correctly: the position of the bar overhead; active shoulders, with the armpits open; tight core and glute muscles; knees tracking over the feet, but not out in front of them, and pressing outwardly, weight on the heels. I wasn't able to get the hip crease below the knee, as the movement prescribes, but I made enough progress that I felt like I had accomplished something.

When a new client comes in, the three CrossFit Elysium coaches compare notes, assessing what sort of shape the person is in and guessing his or her background. Says Chang, "If a new client carries 80 extra pounds on them, it's a good bet that their cardiovascular endurance isn't up to speed. Conversely, if they are a marathon runner, they probably have a good base of aerobic endurance, but they're going to get crushed even by an empty barbell [as was my case]. Other clues are more subtle but they're there if you're observant as a coach." He noted when I did my air squats during the warm-up that my torso would lean forward as I got near parallel. "This told me your flexibility, especially in your posterior chain, was probably compromised. As the strength move for that day was overhead squats, this definitely alerted us to be ready for you and that you may need some help. Of course, we always start people light so we can see any movement issues prior to the weight becoming challenging. If PVC or an empty bar is giving you issues, then we know you're not ready for 95 or 135 pounds."

By Monday, I was sore, really sore. My hamstrings were like electric wires, and my shoulders, abs, quads, and wrists ached. Estrada's advice on this subject: Just keep going to class and work through the soreness.

On Monday, July 4, I walked into my second class and saw this on the whiteboard:

WARM-UP
CF x 1

STRENGTH
Off

MET-CON
"Murph" for time
Run 1 mile
100 pull-ups
200 push-ups
300 squats
Run 1 mile
Start and finish with the run, partition reps as desired.
If you have a 20-lb. weight vest or body armor, wear it.

"Murph" was one of the "Hero WODs," long and difficult CrossFit workouts named after fallen soldiers, law-enforcement officers, and firefighters who were also CrossFitters. Below the workout on the Elysium website, the following history was posted:

In memory of Navy Lieutenant Michael Murphy, 29, of Patchogue, N.Y., who was killed in Afghanistan June 28th, 2005. This workout was one of Mike's favorites and he'd named it "Body Armor." From here on it will be referred to as "Murph" in honor of the focused warrior and great American who wanted nothing more in life than to serve this great country and the beautiful people who make it what it is.

I read through the whole WOD several times, reconsidering my stance on the fundamentals program. Suddenly there seemed to be a lot of good reasons to bypass Murph, go to fundamentals, then take a detour past the gym and to the beer garden, where some of my coworkers were planning to go for July 4 festivities. It actually felt like real gravity pulling me toward this detour. Truth is, I couldn't do more than three pull-ups. This workout called for 97 more pull-ups than that.

This is where the concept of *scaling* comes in, where CrossFit becomes manageable even for newbies who can't execute even one of the exercises. Scaling is not well understood outside CrossFit. If all you knew about CrossFit was what you found out by watching the CrossFit Games or looking at the WODs posted on the CrossFit website, it would be easy to for you to conclude that you didn't have a chance and that CrossFit wasn't for you. But those posted WODs are what Greg Glassman calls the "pointy end of the spear." Scaling is a common solution for many CrossFitters and not just newbies. Maybe you can't run, or maybe you can't do push-ups or pull-ups. The coaches scale down the exercises into what you can do.

Standing there in front of the whiteboard on July 4, contemplating my exit, I knew I was nowhere near being able to do 100 regular pull-ups, let alone what's called a "kipping pull-up" where the athlete channels power from the core muscles to the muscles of the extremities through a whip-like pendulum motion. Kipping pull-ups allow CrossFitters to peel off a dozen or more at a time, and the elite members all seem to gravitate toward butterfly kipping pull-ups. These are hauntingly beautiful to watch, and they make the kipping pull-up seem ridiculously easy (which of course it isn't). Elite CrossFitter (and frequent Games competitor) Chris Spealler has famously done more than 100 pull-ups of the butterfly type in fast succession.

THERE ARE DOZENS OF VIDEOS AND TUTORIALS ON YOUTUBE THAT HAVE BEEN POSTED BY DIFFERENT GYMS AND BY INDIVIDUAL CROSSFITTERS.

Some people don't think kipping pull-ups are "real" pull-ups, and it's true they are easier than regular pull-ups. But they also make your heart feel like it's going to explode. They tax major muscle groups, giving you a full-body training effort instead of only an arms-and-shoulders workout. It's almost impossible to describe the kipping pull-up and the butterfly kipping pull-up—except to say that the athlete seems to be slashing through the air with a body snap and a swinging motion—but there are dozens of videos and tutorials on YouTube that have been posted by different gyms and by individual CrossFitters.

At the time, though, I really couldn't do any type of pull-up. I was given a green industrial-strength band to loop over the bar and hook one foot into, stirrup-like, and, to my surprise and delight, it shot me into the air for each pull-up. It made it feel like I weighed 50 pounds. I could do the other elements of the WOD—push-ups, sit-ups, and running—so this was my one scaling mechanism.

Pacing is another useful tool for a workout like Murph. You could parse a workout any way you wanted—do all 100 pull-ups straight through, then 200 push-ups, then 300 squats. Or you could devise circuits. I ended up doing 10 pull-ups (with the band to help me), 20 push-ups (breaking them up into blasts of 5 when I got tired), and 30 air squats (also broken up). Ultimately, it was a steady rhythm in which I noticed the slowly building fatigue in my muscles as the rounds piled up.

The established athletes in the gym took considerably less than an hour to complete the workout. It took me 1 hour and 7 minutes. Afterward, I went down to the Toronado, ordered a pint of black ale, and went out to the beer garden. It was sunny, and my hands still trembled from the workout. I sipped a beer and stared at a wall. It felt good. My love/hate relationship with CrossFit was beginning.

DOSAGE

My first few days fully exposed me to the "high-dose" medicine that CrossFit purports to deliver. The idea is that the most effective exercise is "constantly varying, high-intensity exercise across broad and modal domains." "Constantly varying" simply means that what you do tomorrow is a lot different from what you did today. The coaches hit you with a wide variety of exercises across the course of a week, a month, or a year. The variance speaks to CrossFit's aim to create general fitness and overall health, with programs designed to sacrifice the needs that a "specialist," like a marathoner or a power lifter, for example, would covet.

"High intensity" is the second key element. There's no doubt that 40 minutes on an elliptical trainer with your heart rate at 120 to 130 beats per minute—that is, in the "aerobic zone"—is a very different experience from the one you get in a 7-minute met-con of heavy kettle-bell swings, box-jumping, and burpees. Halfway through an elliptical-trainer workout, you're usually so bored that you'll watch whatever is on the TV screen in front of you just to take your mind off of the tiresome grind. I've done my time on indoor bikes and treadmills; the boredom is insufferable.

Contrast the halfway point on the cardio machine with the halfway point of the 7-minute met-con. Halfway through the met-con, and you are anything but bored, although you may be looking for the exit signs and promising yourself that you'll never come back. There's a searing ray of discomfort that originates deep in the gut and expands through your chest and heart, lending an ache to every desperate breath that you're struggling to take. You are only halfway through the uncomfortable experience, but you can only think about the next 30 seconds. And then the next 30 seconds after that. Those 7 minutes elicit a sharp physiological response from you.

Exercise physiologist Lon Kilgore has a lot to say on the subject of high-intensity bouts of exercise—and why they have not become more mainstream, despite, he says, having been proven more effective. He is the coauthor of the book *Starting Strength: Basic Barbell Training* with Mark Rippetoe and has an extensive background in Olympic lifting. His introduction to CrossFit came when Rippetoe one day handed him a telephone. On the line was Glassman, who had questions for him. The two talked for 90 minutes, and Kilgore began writing for the *CrossFit Journal* on topics of exercise science.

"I think [Glassman] was happy to have someone objective, not having drunk the Kool-Aid, so to speak, considering the system and its workings," Kilgore told me over an exchange of e-mails. "He wasn't worried that we didn't and don't agree on all things. We agree on enough. I was happy to be able to write about science to people who cared."

As a weight lifting specialist, Kilgore wasn't initially interested in pursuing CrossFit-style training. "I played with a few of the workouts after talking to Greg, but as a weight lifter, I specialize my training to that end, so I didn't immerse myself into the training." Curious, however, he bought some pulse oximeters, a device that measures the rate of oxygenation of the subject's blood, and started playing with depressing blood oxygen content by doing CrossFit workouts. Two years later, he used himself as a guinea pig in a study to see how effective CrossFit training really was in improving a set of physiological and clinical measures.

"The caveat here," he says, "was that I had to work hard enough to drop oxygen saturation more than 4 percent, the critical value of hypoxemia." In other words, he had to climb into the pain cave over and over again. The markers blasted upward. "It was an eye-opening and successful pilot. I had a new appreciation for 'get some, go again' and making 'sweat angels.'"

One of the reasons that Kilgore has been both directly and indirectly involved in the CrossFit community for the past six years, he says, is that it achieves what other exercise and fitness program models do not: rapid and tangible progress. Kilgore reports that he has "used the observations of CrossFit trainees and coaches as a springboard to develop the right questions about exercise adaptation and coaching in my role as an academic."

What most concerns Kilgore about the way most people work out is what he sees as an unnatural distance between the conventional fitness concepts they are using and what has long been known to be more effective. "Interval training," he says,

has been around as an endurance performance enhancement tool for decades, if not centuries. But it has been swept under the rug or pushed into the closet in respect to commercial fitness operations for a very long time. Starting in the forties and fifties, developing into a large movement in the sixties, and persisting to this day, is the concept that the only exercise you need for physical health is long, slow endurance work. The high-profile writings of [Kirk] Cureton, [Kenneth] Cooper, and [Tim] Noakes in the 1960s and 1970s portraying jogging as the only type of exercise needed for fitness development and heart-disease prevention created a great impediment to anyone trying to promote comprehensive fitness methods.

What Kilgore says he finds most surprising is that there has been research data since the 1970s and 1980s demonstrating that interval- and circuit-style training improves cardiovascular fitness and other fitness elements better than long, slow, distance-type training. He cites more recent research as well, including work by Izumi Tabata in Japan, Julien Baker in the United Kingdom, and others. He gives Glassman credit for bringing training practice into line with training research and theory: "Greg Glassman recognized the gap between knowledge and practice and synthesized an approach to training that was not unidimensional, nor the typical low-intensity effort for the duration from 30 to 60 minutes," Kilgore says. "That approach can only work with previously sedentary individuals and only for a few months."

Kilgore sees the business of traditional commercial fitness as falling short of what it could be, and even standing in the way of an athlete's progress. "They market glitz and shiny things that are peripheral to fitness, rather than providing actual progress toward fitness," he says. And even in the realm of public health promotion, according to Kilgore, the active paradigm was built around getting as many people as possible to do the minimum amount of physical activity possible to maintain physical health. "Fitness was not part of the equation, and is still not," he notes.

DOING THINGS DIFFERENTLY

The thing about CrossFit, too, is that it's hard. I quickly began to see what used to be relatively benign pieces of strength equipment in a new light; just being near some of them started to give me low-grade anxiety. Take an innocuous rowing machine, the Concept2 ergometer. Over the past 20 years, I had hopped on rowing machines now and again, usually when some machine or other was being occupied. My one memory of them: boring. I'd commit to using the rowing machine for 15 minutes and would barely make that, not because of overexertion, but because of underexcitement.

One day on the WOD whiteboard, the met-con was a 500-meter row. Fine, I thought. I had covered that several times over in rowing sessions of yore. But as I listened to Estrada's explanation of our task, I found out there was a catch: This was a time-trial, and you had to go all-out. The point was to find out how fast you could row the 500 meters.

"We have a quick and simple one today," Estrada said, announcing the met-con. "The trick to this is to go out as hard as you can and hold on for as long as you can." We went in heats, four of us at a time. So you could feel the race over your shoulder (even though, of course, no one moved an inch).

STILL, I KEPT GOING BACK. MORE AND MORE, IT WAS BECAUSE I BEGAN TO GET TO KNOW THE OTHERS.

When Estrada said "Go," we all went at the machines like we were trying to save the *Titanic*. Estrada would shout out comments containing two types of information during the flurry. If he saw someone dogging it, he got on that individual, telling him or her to push harder. He also gave out technique tips. The chief mistake that he pointed out was failure to use the legs and core sufficiently in the first phase of the pull stroke. By 150 meters, the brain begins to send out signals that it doesn't like what you're up to. The first wave of discomfort rolls in. It steadily gets worse. By 300 meters, the arms don't work as well as they used to. The chest heaves for air. Lactic acid begins to pull in key areas. The last 100 meters, provided you have followed Estrada's instructions, get fuzzy. You can't help but slow down a bit, and all of us were making odd suffering noises. I hit 500 meters in 1:34. That's all it took in terms of time. It seemed much longer. We all wobbled off of the machines and walked in circles or fell to the floor. I tasted metal in my mouth and coughed for the next few hours. "CrossFit Lung," it's called. I will never again underestimate a rowing machine.

Because of moments like this, in July, August, and September I woke up every day that I had to do CrossFit feeling nervous about it. I knew I would be in the middle of a met-con later that day, maybe at the three-minute mark of an eight-minute workout, feeling sorry for myself because the next five minutes were going to punish me.

Still, I kept going back. More and more, it was because I began to get to know the others. There was Miriam, who always sang my name when I came in;

Brian, an elite soldier in the navy who went back and forth from combat missions in Afghanistan; Irene, the inspirational leader of Elysium who always gave me a hug; Sam, always wearing low-top Converse shoes and a Toronado T-shirt; Briana, sleepy-eyed because she worked graveyard shifts and went to grad school, but attacked workouts with ferocity; Karla and Dave, two of the gym's "Firebreathers" (see Chapter 8), who always showed up early, worked hard, and stayed afterward in their impassioned pursuit of excellence. And a host of others.

The accountability factor ensured by the whiteboard also certainly had something to do with me showing up four or five times per week. But mostly, it was because I knew these guys were showing up, and I liked their company and the sense of community. I knew how guilty I'd feel if I wasn't there to endure it with them.

But I was also getting results, and, most surprisingly, in an area CrossFit terms "mobility." I hadn't been mobile since I was 17. I was about to get a lot of it back by first doing what Kelly Starrett, the CrossFit movement guru, calls "making the invisible visible."

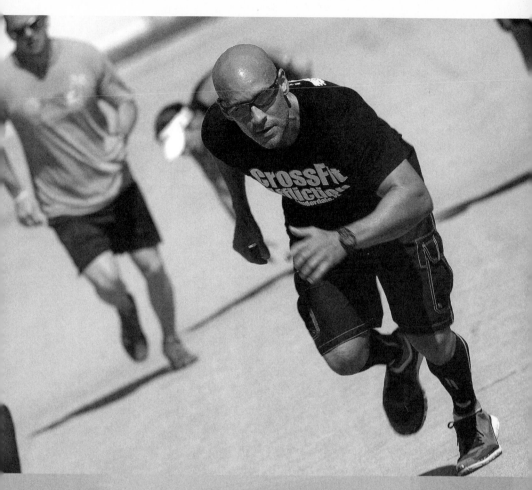

MAKING THE INVISIBLE VISIBLE

4

CROSSFIT'S FOCUS ON MOVEMENT AND MOBILITY

CROSSFIT HAS AN OBSESSION WITH MOVEMENT. MOST PEOPLE WHO HAVE HEARD of it, but who have not yet tried it, have the impression that it is a daredevil version of exercise that is all about and only about maximum heart rate and pushing till you puke. But what is drilled into your head in class, in special sessions, and in certification programs are the basics of movement and a religious intensity for mastering movement technique. How you pick something up off the ground, move it, and put it back down—the way you would when loading a bag of grain from the ground onto a trailer—or how you complete your pull-up, in case you ever find yourself dangling from a cliff and have to pull yourself to safety, is the all-important focus. So it's not so much daredevil as it is functional—sort of like when your mom taught you how to cross the street, but as if she also taught you, at the same time, what to do if you suddenly found an 18-wheeler barreling toward you when you were out in the middle of the road.

This intense focus on functional movement is one of CrossFit's defining characteristics and sets it well apart from how one might be taught to train at a typical fitness center. Most CrossFit WODs are organized around either the essential functional movements—deadlifts, squats, Olympic lifts, pull-ups, push-ups—or variations of the essential movements. In the case of squats, you might be asked to perform back squats, front squats, overhead squats, air squats, and so forth.

Greg Glassman says to look at the functional movements from which CrossFit draws its inspiration and compare these with the isolated movements that weight machines allow. The former movements (deadlifts, box jumps, running, rowing, and muscle-ups, for example), are compound. They employ many muscle groups; can exhaust you; resemble motions that are natural and can be seen at construction sites, on farms, or in disaster rescue operations; and build in the athlete a unique capacity to move large loads relatively long distances in short spurts of time. The latter (curl machines, leg extensions, lateral raises, and the like) have none of these virtues, and because they aren't natural, Glassman argues, they can do more harm than good. He points to the knee extension as an example, saying that the way the machine has you work your leg, the patella tendon doesn't sit properly in its groove.

Glassman imported his reverence for skilled compound movements like those existing in gymnastics and Olympic lifting into the world of CrossFit. This DNA permeates the spectrum of CrossFit's movement choreography. And the discussion is always being nudged forward by new voices and perspectives.

THE MOVEMENT OF MOVEMENT

I attended a CrossFit Level 1 coaching certification seminar in Austin, Texas, led by senior CFHQ trainer Todd Widman, in December 2011. The seminar covered everything within the CrossFit model, from nutrition to programming, and also put the attendees through CrossFit workouts. But the bulk of the time was spent on learning how to teach the foundational movements in a lecture/lab combination format. I saw, for example, a highly detailed talk and demonstration of proper squat mechanics. Instruction followed, with students split into groups and each group assigned a seminar trainer. My group was assigned Lindsey Smith, one of the top CrossFit athletes in the world.

Smith had us stand in a circle while she taught us the basic mechanics and "cues" of how to perform the air squat correctly. She also taught us how to teach others the air squat. I got pulled into the middle of the circle because Smith immediately identified a flaw in my technique. She pressed the group to teach me how to do it right—they had to identify the flaw and advise me on how to correct it.

We went through this sequence with other primary functional movements in CrossFit as well. The push-press (I again got pulled into the middle); the push jerk (more time in the middle); the snatch (pulled into the middle); the clean and jerk (they saw I was getting really annoyed and decided not to pull me into the middle again). We also had sessions on how to properly perform a kipping pull-up and a muscle-up.

Movement is a huge component of another specialty focus within CrossFit: endurance. The endurance program is CrossFit's answer to running and triathlon. I attended a weekend seminar in Hermosa Beach, California, that was led by Brian MacKenzie, who is built like a strong safety. He is heavily inked, with his tattoos ranging from an owl on his back to an all-black sleeve tattoo, to go with his black hair. He conducts heavy experimentation with his diet, most of it grass-fed beef. For carbs, he prefers garden vegetables ground to a fine powder with a food processor.

MacKenzie's path to ultramarathoning, Ironman triathlon, and CrossFit came after a phase in his early twenties when he realized "when I get bored I get destructive." He found a channel for burning off excess energy in a dilapidated indoor cycling gym in Orange County. The classes were so hard, MacKenzie told me, that they forced him to find a spiritual path. The path took him further into the otherworld of crushingly painful endurance workouts. Spinning led to triathlon, running races, and Ironmans as well as to 100-mile trail races, which he said nearly destroyed him. "I would be on the couch for a week after an ultra. But I love 100-mile runs," he says. "I love the place you have to go to when you're up against it in an ultra."

He soon started to experiment with ways to do long races without feeling completely beat afterward. He studied with the Pose Method running scientist and guru Dr. Nicholas Romanov, and he also came across CrossFit. He was soon hooked. He embraced the utility concepts of high-intensity exercise as a foundation-building mechanism for endurance sport, eventually opening up a CrossFit gym. He sampled mixes of CrossFit, running, power lifting, and a method of programming that was antithetical to conventional periodization strategies. MacKenzie also experimented with the conclusions produced by the high-intensity exercise studies of Nishimura Tabata that indicated there were high-end endurance benefits to be had with short bursts of anaerobic intervals with short recoveries.

THE ENDURANCE PROGRAM IS CROSSFIT'S ANSWER TO RUNNING AND TRIATHLON.

MacKenzie would crank a treadmill's incline to 12 percent and run the intervals so hard that he would black out. He conducted similar experiments with recovery techniques (including using a jackhammer-like sports massage device he built from a pneumatic nail gun), nutrition, and hydration. The end result was that he was able to create a physiological infrastructure that could absorb the brutality of a 20-hour trail race. He extended his experiments into a coaching forum and applied his findings to triathlon, becoming the endurance specialty seminar leader for CrossFit. He now has a loyal following around the world of runners and triathletes who use his methods.

During the weekend seminar in Hermosa Beach, his lectures focused on endurance, but they were broken up by movement skill sessions. These consisted of Pose running drills across the parking lot—correcting faulty footstrikes, learning proper arm movement, exchanging long strides for high-rep rates of turnover. He teaches runners how to develop the "hollow rock" body position—a posture borrowed from the gymnastics world that allows flows of energy to move from the core of the body outward. He talks about powering your run from the hamstrings and glutes instead of the quads and hip flexors.

MacKenzie and his coaches watched us run and helped us tweak our styles. Over and over, he would grab my foot as I tried to simulate the piston-like, hamstring-powered pumping motion of the Pose technique, and he would show me the correct pattern. Over and over he would remind people to activate their core muscles to about 30 percent, and learn how to do it in a way that didn't mess up their breathing. Position, movement, position, movement. That was the heart of the CrossFit endurance seminar.

Another specialty seminar with movement at its heart was the CrossFit Olympic-lifting session led by Mike Burgener. Burgener is a former competitive Olympic lifter, a USA Olympic-lifting coach, and a former U.S. Marine and Notre Dame football player; he has also taught San Diego grade-school kids the complex movements that make up the clean and jerk and the snatch. He thus has an interesting background to bring to the gym when he teaches greenhorn CrossFit crowds. He displays a mastery for getting a group's attention and keeping it tuned in. He uses fear, too—fear of burpees. If Burgener says the word "burpees" at any time during the seminar and the group doesn't respond, with Marine-recruit-like passion, by shouting, "YEAH, BURPEES!!" then the group gets to do an onslaught of burpees. From the get-go, Burgener tries to trip up the group, solidifying a keen level of attention as he then swoops in and teaches the students how to teach others. He covers how to warm up, how to do "skill transfer exercises," how to snatch, how to jerk, and how to use footwork, movement, speed, and position. Everything is broken down into simplified pieces: positions, and movements from positions. Movement, mobility, and more movement.

But the CrossFit obsession with movement is perhaps personified best by Kelly Starrett.

THE MAN BEHIND CROSSFIT MOBILITY

Kelly Starrett is a physical therapist, a CrossFit box owner, and a former national-class kayaker. Within the context of CrossFit's fixation on movement, you might say he is super-obsessed. And his obsession is packaged along with charisma and a unique talent for coaching. He has attracted a global audience through his website, MobilityWOD.com, in which he plays a sort of run-and-gun offense with his ideas and insights on movement in more than 400 short instructional videos. He has been hired to teach seminars or train with a wide variety of groups, including U.S. Navy SEALs, U.S. Army Special Forces, the San Francisco Ballet, Tour de France-level cyclists, world-record powerlifters, and Olympic-medalist rowers.

Starrett and his wife, Juliet, opened San Francisco CrossFit in 2005. His expertise in coaching movement stems from having worked as a physical therapist (PT) at the highly respected Stone Clinic in San Francisco as well as from thousands of hours spent coaching at the gym. His current PT practice is in fact located at the gym. On weekends, he conducts CrossFit mobility seminars around the country, bringing his convictions on the subjects of rehab, injury prevention, and the triangular relationship between movement, power, and performance to his audiences.

Starrett doesn't just coach mobility, though; he lives it. He doesn't just preach about how sitting in an office chair all day messes you up; he owns a desk that requires you to stand. He doesn't take his flexibility for granted, either. As a member of the U.S. Canoe and Kayak team, he had his career cut short by neck pain that was so severe he couldn't turn his head sideways. And he wasn't able to run more than 100 yards until he got deep into the study of movement.

Watch Starrett in the midst of overseeing operations at SFCF, and you'll inevitably see him practicing one of the major concepts that he preaches: Bury stretching and mobility work into your day. Starrett will lower into a deep squat, holding it for long periods of time and making it look as comfortable as if he were sinking into a La-Z-Boy. Or he'll take a band of industrial-grade rubber, loop it around a pull-up bar, and begin "flossing," as he calls it, the deep-seated clumps of tightness in his shoulder, back, and neck that more likely than not came from a heavy powerlifting workout or 20-minute met-con.

Starrett launched MobilityWOD.com in August 2010 after hopping on a skateboard and filming himself with an iPhone. In the ensuing year, he posted videos almost daily. It's clear from the videos that Starrett has a lot of criticism for the way sports medicine is traditionally practiced—he feels that the injured runner, for example, can get trapped in a quagmire of high-priced and unnecessary treatments that may not even be effective. What may annoy him most about the way sports medicine is often practiced is that it puts the responsibility for health in the hands of the provider as opposed to the athlete. The tagline on MobilityWOD.com reads:

> This blog is intended as a jump-off point for athletes to systematically begin to address their nasty tissues and grody joint mobility. Use at your own risk and stop if you think it's gonna hurt you, your spine is going to come out your throat, or your face goes numb. But, understand that you should be responsible for your own business. Don't wait until you need a new knee. Pony up.

Once upon a time, not very long ago, I was the guy who was close to needing a new knee. And Starrett was a key part of my first foray into CrossFit.

FIRST MEETING

I first met Starrett in late 2010. As I looked for San Francisco CrossFit, I was experiencing a few final minutes of walking via a zombie-like technique, gaining most of my propulsion from my overburdened left leg so that I could step down as lightly as possible with my right foot. It hurt. For weeks, I had been taking Advil and applying ice, trying to get the pain to retreat, but with no effect. The knee kept buckling beneath me. The injury was just getting worse, and it was getting weirder.

I was near Crissy Field in the Presidio, which lines the bay just east of the Golden Gate Bridge, and the bridge, lit into glory in the midmorning sun, was right in my face. I followed a path around a former U.S. Army commissary that had been turned into a massive sporting-goods store.

According to Google Maps, SFCF was at the Sports Basement. I had looked inside the store and couldn't find anything, so I figured maybe the box was in a building out back. The path led to a northside parking lot and a fenced gate. I walked through the gate and saw just what you'd expect to find behind a Walmart-sized sporting-goods store: big Dumpsters, a row of sea kayaks, docking platforms for incoming trucks, and storage containers. I was baffled. But then my eyes caught something in one corner of the parking lot, underneath a highway overpass. It turned out to be several people in gym clothes, lifting weights and hopping onto boxes. I had found SFCF.

The closest things to walls at SFCF are the intersecting lines created by storage containers. Two of the containers are packed with weights, barbells, rowing ergometers, and other training equipment. The third container is empty except for a massage table and a side stand, with, among a few other odds and ends, a multicolored dog toy. This, as I found out, is Kelly Starrett's PT office.

Starrett thinks of the CrossFit gym as a lab in which the good coach should be spotting flaws, or "holes," in the mechanics of a CrossFitter. If the holes are left unchecked, they will eventually become the reason why a runner needs a knee replacement, or a ballet star needs Achilles' tendon surgery, or a tennis player has to quit because she blows out her back. If they're caught early enough, though, new fitness techniques can be instituted, stopping the problem in its tracks and preventing injury.

Because of Starrett, San Francisco CrossFit has become a think tank on movement and athletics. Starrett sketches out Venn diagrams and deep flow-chart-style explanations. These speak of the "rich complexity" that takes place as a CrossFit athlete progresses from a fundamentals class to the intermediate and advanced levels of CrossFit. These progressions translate into methods for getting the postsurgery athlete healthy and back on his feet. Starrett calls it the "Hierarchy of Movement." The *CrossFit Journal* archives dozens of Starrett lecture videos in which he criticizes the overall business of sports-medicine clinics and the way they suck money out of people. He believes that "all human beings should be able to perform basic maintenance on themselves."

STARRETT THINKS OF THE CROSSFIT GYM AS A LAB IN WHICH THE GOOD COACH SHOULD BE SPOTTING FLAWS, OR "HOLES," IN THE MECHANICS OF A CROSSFITTER.

I was here, and I was going to put this particular Starrett conviction to the test.

I was thoroughly prepared to give him a detailed report on the condition of my knee, both past and present, and to explain how the injury occurred, the nuances of when and where the pain struck when I took a step, and everything I could conjure up to help him help me. I also wanted him to get a distinct sense of the level of my desperation. This had been step one whenever I'd consulted with any doctor or medical specialist about any injury.

Starrett never gave me a chance to deliver my little presentation. The first thing he did was walk me to a spot on the rubber matting of the SFCF flooring, where he had me stand with my feet a little wider than shoulder-width apart.

SFCF resembles the kind of camouflaged tactical station you'd expect in an army headquarters operation in the field. I was facing a large whiteboard with various CrossFit scrawlings on it, including times, met-con information, and stick-man drawings with arrows pointed at joints and alignments. The equipment around me fit in with this image: a metal monkey-bar-like apparatus, glute-ham developer devices, a beer keg, a grill, and a spherical cement rock. Starrett asked me to do a deep-knee bend—a squat, as far as I could go. As I did what he asked, his eyes followed the track of my knees. Starrett gleaned almost everything he needed to know about my knees from the pattern of movement—the track of my knees, the position of my spine, and the depth I was able to manage.

WHAT'S IN A SQUAT?

The squat is a key to the CrossFit universe, and Starrett is one of a number of select experts whose insight into movement and biomechanics helps to direct the main themes of the greater CrossFit discussion. Greg Glassman, too, places high value on the squat. In the well of the *CrossFit Journal*, an early video of Glassman shows him teaching a clinic on the air squat—a squat performed without any additional weight.

Glassman argues that being able to squat correctly is vital to a fulfilling existence as a functionally moving human being. The squat, with or without load, according to Glassman, is a powerful example of what functional movement is. And a functional movement, he says, is vastly superior to the isolated one-muscle movements found in traditional gyms. A squat is a multijoint movement tapping a universal motor-recruitment pattern; it brings muscle groups throughout the body into action and therefore allows a person to move a large load a significant distance in an efficient, powerful way. A leg-extension machine, in contrast, isolates the muscles on the front of the leg; it is thus inefficient, if not unnatural, and it does not increase one's capacity to move weight in any sort of powerful or meaningful way.

One of the most common warnings issued within the world of weight train-ing is that if you're going to squat, or use a leg-press-type machine, you should not go below a 90-degree angle with the knee. You are warned that this will grind up your knees; you'll be carted off for orthopedic surgery. Glassman argues that these warnings are ridiculous and that being able to perform a squat where the crease of the hip descends deeper than the line of the knees is crucial. It not only increases a person's CrossFit performance but is beneficial for overall health and quality of life. Glassman argues that a squat is an example of functional movement—a movement that allows a human being to move large loads of weight a long distance with good speed. Functional movement is a movement, Glassman says, that a human being uses with optimal power and efficiency to perform work. Squats, deadlifts, rowing, and pull-ups all are examples of functional movements that Glassman says can be identified in real tasks that must be done in the blue-collar world. Getting 100 bales of hay onto a truck, for example, is most efficiently accomplished by using the clean and jerk.

"The squat is essential to your well-being," Glassman wrote in the *CrossFit Journal* in December 2002. "The squat can both greatly improve your athleticism and keep your hips, back, and knees sound and functioning in your senior years. Not only is the squat not detrimental to the knees[...] it is remarkably rehabilitative of cranky, damaged, or delicate knees. In fact, if you do not squat, your knees are not healthy regardless of how free of pain or discomfort you are. This is equally true of the hips and back."

But why should a runner, for example, care about being able to perform a full squat? For one thing, when you run you're performing countless numbers of quarter-depth, one-legged squats, though you never flex and extend the leg as you do in a full squat. Glassman, Starrett, and MacKenzie would say that if you're unable to perform a full squat with good technique—flat back, knees tracking over the feet, hip crease below the line of the knees—you're "leaving performance on the table," as Starrett puts it. In other words, failure to develop the full squat means you're not availing your body of all of the athletic potential waiting to be claimed for it. Of course, you can shoot with an M16 and hit the target from 10 feet away, a Glassman analogy goes, but where you really flush out your weaknesses is when you try and hit the target from 300 feet.

This is what Kelly Starrett would later tell me is the idea behind making "the invisible visible"—using CrossFit-style training to see where the lurking weaknesses are before they manifest themselves into injuries. A runner with the mobility and strength to perform lots of air squats consistently with proper technique is going to have more to draw from, especially in the depths of a long, hard race, than the broken runner who can't squat down to save his life. When you can't squat, Starrett says, there's a hidden problem that will one day work its way to the surface.

At the time I performed the first air squat of my life under the eye of Kelly Starrett, I had no idea what he was doing or why my form on a squat mattered.

It was new to me to be consulting with physical therapists, sports doctors, and the like.

Squat? No problem, I thought. In high-school football, I had done them all the time, with a barbell loaded to 300 pounds on my shoulders. Usually it was half or quarter squats back then. Starrett directed me to try and go as deep as possible without any weight at all. He watched the lumbar spine, the arch, the split between the frontal plane of my body and the rear plane, and the center of mass—the plumb line splitting the two planes. He looked for hip flexion and extension and midline stabilization. He watched to see whether my heels were coming off the ground (they were), whether I dropped my head (I did), and whether my knees rolled inward (they did)—all three considered faults. If I were to get underneath an Olympic bar loaded with a few 45-pound weights on either end to do these things, I could do the sort of damage that has physicians and chiropractors warning people off from squats.

He never even asked me which knee was bothering me. After watching me attempt the air squat, he started instructing me in how to do it properly. His focus was on teaching me how to keep my knees from rolling inward and how to keep them from moving out beyond an imaginary vertical plane rising from my feet. I had a flashback to the one ballet class I'd taken in my life, in 1984 at the University of Iowa, where I was taught how to do a *grand plie* by a former Joffrey Ballet dancer, who corrected me by swatting me with a pink ballet shoe. Starrett's method of correcting my movement path was a bit different: "Break this plane and you owe me a beer," he said. I could barely do what he was asking, and I didn't have a drop of extra weight loaded onto my shoulders.

GAS-O BRAKE-O

The hour I spent with Starrett was a high-speed indoctrination into his philosophy. After the squat clinic, I went into the PT office, and Starrett proceeded to test the range of motion in both of my knees. He had me extend and flex my legs and added pressure to see how far they could go. My right knee had considerably less range than my left.

"Are you okay with that?" he asked.

"Uh...no?"

It was not a question I had ever considered. I had come to believe that my lack of flexibility with the right knee was simply a given. Starrett then reached over to the side table and picked up the one tool he appeared to have in his storage-container office. He held it in the air and said, "Dog toy." He then began to use it around the kneecap like he was opening a beer bottle with it. No ultrasound, no muscle stimulator. Just a three-dollar chunk of rubber plucked from a PetCo bin.

"I went to Mexico once and rented a car and abused it, playing 'Gas-o, Brake-o,'" he said. "To play Gas-o, Brake-o, I kept the gas pedal pegged to the floor and accelerated and decelerated with the brake. Wham! I'm redlining. Until the car is about to blow up. So I swing into my hotel and park the car and a guy comes running out and says, 'Señor!,' pointing at the rear tire because it's erupted into flames. If you're a runner with really tight hips and poor sliding surfaces in your joints, you're running around revving your engine with the brakes on. You're playing Gas-o, Brake-o. And now your knee is on fire."

ONE OF STARRETT'S PRIMARY TECHNIQUES: HE ADVISES ATHLETES TO WORK BOTH ABOVE AND BELOW A PROBLEM AREA.

Starrett told me that the fire within my knee was such that my body basically shut it down to stop me from pushing it any further. He then told me that it was my job to take care of this. Yes, he said, you need to see a doctor when you have a weird pain or injury, to make certain it's not a pathology or disease disguised as an annoying sports-injury pain. But once you're clear, you can take care of yourself.

"You cut your finger and you know what to do—you clean it up and put on the Band-Aid. Why not be able to work with your muscle tissue? You can take care of your body in a way that will minimize injury risk and boost your performance until you're 110 years old. Bam! World domination."

He taught me two stretches and told me to practice them often. I was to hold each stretch for two minutes. One was a painful position that had me kneeling with one foot stepping forward and the other leg folded up behind me with the knee planted on the ground. Holding the position for two minutes was time spent in what Starrett called "the pain tunnel." But when I stood up again, I could feel a change in how the front of my right thigh felt in relation to my knee. The hip flexor had been thoroughly loosened up. Starrett also had me do a long, deep, calf-muscle stretch. These two stretches, the calf and the hip flexor, gave me a concrete example of what I later learned is one of Starrett's primary techniques: He advises athletes to work both above and below a problem area.

My session with Starrett had lasted only an hour. I had been limping for six weeks before the start of the appointment. And the limp had disappeared.

GROWING PAINS?

Some CrossFit ringleaders suspect that as the CrossFit community grows, a lack of focus on quality movement may be leaking in. They seem set to counter the problem, however, and that is why seminars and certifications have become such an important part of the mission.

The number of CrossFitters has exploded in the past five years. Too many CrossFitters too fast, too many new gyms, and insufficient oversight by CrossFit HQ could, theoretically, put the concept of virtuosity—the mastery of essential skills—at risk. At least, that is the fear. And since CrossFit is not a franchise system, it could be seen as lacking the quality controls typical of franchise businesses. The affiliate system allows for a great deal of flexibility and interpretation, and that can be a strength, but this same flexibility makes it inevitable that a few bad gyms will be in the mix.

Anecdotal reports of high injury rates in CrossFit are linked not only to this lack of control and the rapid growth of the sport but also to the number of new coaches being certified in weekend seminars and launched into the world. Another concern is that, with ESPN broadcasting the CrossFit Games, they will be viewed by more people, and the emphasis of CrossFit will seem to be on how fast athletes can do a workout, how much they can lift, or both, instead of how well they are performing the movements. Performing the movements well equates to performing them safely, so if this shift trickles down to CrossFit box coaches and the way they train their clients, this is definitely a problem. At the elite level, sponsorships and financial rewards could exacerbate the situation. If this trickle-down theory is correct, stories of injuries will multiply. CrossFit will be pegged as an injury machine, and the stories will scare newcomers away.

At the CrossFit Level 1 seminar in Austin, I saw the following written on a chalkboard: "CrossFit is not the CrossFit Games." The new coaches were being encouraged to take this message back to their affiliates and reinforce the principles of virtuosity-the mission of giving one's attention to the mastery of skill.

The weekend I went to Austin, five other Level 1 certification classes were in progress. Each had about 30 people in attendance. Not everyone took the test to become a certified coach. (I didn't, for example, and I know there were others who came simply to learn more about CrossFit.) Still, the pace of producing coaches in CrossFit is high. Consider that the first coaching certification was held December 2-4, 2002, and it was taught by Greg Glassman with two attendees. In 2011, according to CrossFit HQ, 14,593 people attended Level 1 coaching certification training.

STARRETT ON MOBILITY:
WHY CROSSFIT IS A FREAK FOR MOVEMENT

Kelly Starrett, a spokesman for movement and mobility in CrossFit, explained to me why mechanics are such a big deal in the quest for fitness and athleticism.

The greatest expression of force generated and controlled by the body, he said, comes from the hips. Second is the shoulders. In running, for example, faulty hip mechanics lead to a loss of potential explosive power, which should come from the hips, and a transition to an emphasis on the smaller muscles of the extremities, such as the quadriceps.

Dysfunction in the hips or shoulders can thus lead to injuries in the extremities. Weakness and imbalance in the hips or shoulders will place inappropriate stress on other musculoskeletal structures further down the chain. The knees, ankles, feet, wrists, hamstrings, and calves are especially vulnerable. This can turn into an ugly cycle of chronic injury. Indeed, the more motivated the athlete is, the worse the problem gets: Because the highly motivated athlete has a psychological determination to perform, her body will reroute power around old joint and tissue injuries and just keep going, but with a suboptimal chain of power, weak links, and weak range of motion. All of this saps power and performance, ultimately leading to breakdown.

The ideal flow of power is from the core muscles of the body to the extremities. With the body properly organized in a neutral position, an athlete will channel more force from the hips and the shoulders into propulsion. Starrett says to think of the human body as a machine the way an engineer thinks of a motorcycle or a rocket. An engineer wouldn't leave efficiency to chance; nor should the CrossFitter.

Taking the time to perfect positioning, movement, and technique is worth it because it will enable you to develop the most powerful and efficient motor-recruitment patterns possible. With the mastery of movement, you can make the most of your muscles and find out what they have to offer. The better prepared you are in this domain, the more you'll be able to meet the challenges of a hard effort when you begin to redline or face muscular exhaustion. The more efficient you can be in all situations, the more you have saved up for the final miles or minutes of an effort.

The key to achieving an optimal flow of power from the core to the extremities is midline stabilization. Starrett will ask a client to put out her arm and imagine that the elbow is the trunk of her body. So try it. With the muscles of the arm relaxed, what sort of brace can you make with the arm? Chances are, if you haven't done this before, that you can make practically no brace at all. With a neutral spine, organized into a stiff trunk by engaging the core muscles into what's referred to as "midline stabilization," however, overextension and underextension can be prevented. "Think of a rigid spine as a big lever arm. With a stiff trunk you can recruit the muscles of the hips and the muscles of the shoulders more efficiently," Starrett told me. Your main draw of power then comes from the most powerful muscles; extremities pitch in down the line.

If you don't have full range of motion in a joint, you're opening yourself up to injury. You're preventing yourself from reaching higher levels of performance, too. If you lose hip control, or shoulder control, you're going to be vulnerable to injury; it's as simple as that. People often think they have a wrist problem or an ankle problem when what they really have is a shoulder problem or a hip problem. When a knee hurts, or a wrist is destroyed, the problem just may be related to the fact that the athlete can't do a body-weight squat without collapsing his spine.

If you have limited range of motion, it's costing you—so try to fix it. "Let's say you're missing 20 percent of your posterior range of motion," Starrett says. "First off, how much energy does it cost you just to be you? If you open up that hip, the cost will go down. Being efficient costs less. It frees up more energy to be put in other places."

Is that a problem? Maybe not. I came away from the certification training feeling like it was pretty thorough. The information was solid and well presented, and a lot was packed into the two days in terms of both lectures and activities. I don't know what they could have done to make it better. The way I saw it, CrossFit was to a certain extent in the hands of the future coaches themselves. When I looked at the rows of my classmates, I didn't think Todd Widman and

CFHQ necessarily had to be responsible for whether these now-certified coaches truly became good at coaching. The truly great CrossFit coaches are ultimately going to be self-made—they're going to have to have the talent and work ethic to do a difficult thing well.

The key for CrossFitters, especially those who are new to it, is to find the coaches who have succeeded in doing that.

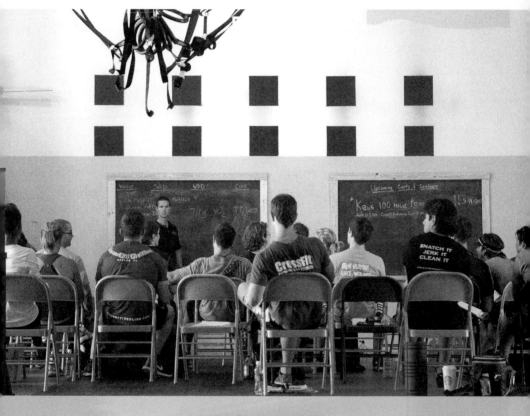

TWO OARS IN THE WATER

5

CROSSFIT'S ONE-TWO PUNCH OF DIET AND EXERCISE

IN MY FIRST MONTH AT CROSSFIT ELYSIUM, THE GYM'S MEMBERS TOOK PART IN a local CrossFit competition held at a neighboring box. I'd seen the CrossFit Games, but I'd never been to one of these smaller competitions. One of the participating CrossFit Elysium members was Briana Drost, a 25-year-old police dispatcher who worked night shifts. During the day, she was earning a master's degree in psychology. So it was that when she came to work out at the gym, which she managed several days a week, she was a little bleary-eyed. Nevertheless, she seemed to relish beating me in workouts. Tired as she must have been after pulling a shift prior to a workout, she invariably turned on her fierce inner warrior when she was there, giving every workout all she had—and flashing me her slightly carnivorous smile whenever she proved herself able to outdo me, a fairly common occurrence.

At the competition, I got a chance to watch Briana's moxie. The competition consisted of three different workouts spread over the course of a brick-oven-hot Saturday in San Diego. The WOD I watched her do was a mix of kettle-bell high pulls, burpees, front squats, and kettle-bell swings, all within a 12-minute time cap. The first to finish would be the winner, so rest between sets and reps was as unwanted as it was wanted. The gym was packed with members of the three participating boxes, a rabid audience lining the competition space. It reminded me of a high-school wrestling tournament where the spectators are red-faced and screaming at the athletes as they suffer on the center mat. It was standing-room-only, unless you wanted to sit on a stack of bumper weights.

Briana was lashing her way through the noise with a 35-pound kettle bell as two of the three Elysium coaches, Leon Chang and Paul Estrada, kept up their style of scream-coaching to push her as hard as possible. She permitted herself a few short breaks, her fists on her hip bones, her face cherry red as she took in air. Chang and Estrada would shout brief instructions, essentially to get her moving again, never allowing her to linger past three or so breaths.

Briana struck me as a total athlete—lean, strong, committed, and driven. I assumed she had always been this way, that it was a case of CrossFit being a magnet for someone with a hard-core personality type who was seeking an outlet. But then she shared a "before" picture with me, showing what she had looked like when she'd first started CrossFit, and an "after" picture taken a year later.

I experienced a jolt of surprise. The "before" Briana was tired, heavy, and clearly suffering the ill effects of a 12-hour graveyard shift as a police dispatcher. "I was working 40 hours a week, chained to a desk," she told me. "And I was in my first year of graduate school, studying psychology. I wasn't eating well or exercising. I was tired of feeling tired all the time. The scale was reading 159 pounds—I'd gained 30. What had I done?" She had seen friends achieve significant transformations after training with CrossFit, and she asked them, "'Oh my god. What is it exactly that you are doing?'" Drost decided to join CrossFit Elysium in August 2010.

Her own results just a year later were as significant as what she had seen her friends achieve. But as Briana would later detail for me, what exactly they were doing was not just CrossFit; there was another component that she put into practice as she learned from them. The fastest ascent from fat to fit for her, she said, occurred when she put into place CrossFit's emphasis on nutrition.

NUTRITION: THE BEDROCK OF CROSSFIT

Per the CrossFit pyramid model, nutrition is the bedrock, the foundation, of the CrossFit way of life. This emphasis is opposed to the way distance runners often think of food. It's not uncommon to hear a runner say, "I run so I can eat anything I want." Documented thoroughly within articles and videos archived in the *CrossFit Journal* is the position that without the right nutrition, CrossFitters will receive only a fraction of the possible benefits of CrossFit. In her first few months of doing CrossFit, Drost didn't bother changing her eating habits. She loved Denny's Grand Slams, food-stand beef chimichangas, and assorted other junk. And she noticed that although her body composition and overall fitness were responding to the work, the reading on the scale hadn't budged.

In videos of Greg Glassman answering questions at the 2011 CrossFit Games, he speaks on the subject of diet. "Excessive consumption of refined carbohydrate is the real 800-pound gorilla of metabolic derangement that is killing Americans by millions," he said, referring to the relationship between poor diet and insulin resistance, adult-onset diabetes, heart disease, and cancer. It was only natural for CrossFit to apply nutritional principles, since its ultimate aim was to define and generate improved health. But Glassman also spoke about a direct correlation between improved diet and improved performance. He cited a number of reasons for this connection, including the benefits of fat loss and muscle gain.

"A guy drops 20 pounds of blubber and picks up 5 pounds of muscle, there's a 15 pound differentiation on the scale, he's got 10 more pull-ups," Glassman said. He added that a CrossFitter has only "one oar in the water if you're talking about nutrition or only one oar in the water if you're talking about movement." The combination of a high-performance diet and CrossFit training, he noted, can move you into the "jet stream of adaptation." And adaptation, for Glassman, is what improvement in athletic performance is all about.

COMBINING THE PALEO AND ZONE DIETS

In CrossFit, a healthy diet is two-dimensional. First is the quality of the food you eat, which has to do with "the paleo diet." A cursory sweep through the websites of CrossFit gyms will easily produce paleo recipes and several links to paleo diet websites.

At its essence, the paleo diet suggests that by evolutionary standards, our bodies are still more in sync with how we ate more than 10,000 years ago than with the way we have been eating since the dawn of the agricultural and industrial ages. Paleolithic people were hunters and gatherers. They ate meat and vegetables, nuts and seeds, some fruit, very little starch, and virtually no sugar (aside from the occasional honey stolen from bees). Agricultural development started to change all this, and the change was for the worse, say paleo diet enthusiasts. Eat a strict paleo diet, and you will be eating mostly meat, poultry, fish, vegetables, nuts, and fruit and avoiding the likes of pasta, bread, milk, and cheese.

"It's the perimeter of the grocery store," Glassman says, meaning stick to the meat and produce sections, and it will be hard to go wrong. "If it has a food label on it? It's not food. You don't see food labels on the chicken, tomatoes, apples, pears, oranges." This is advice that's essential "for avoiding heart disease, death, and misery," as Glassman puts it.

Working in concert with the paleolithic diet for CrossFit is the popular Zone Diet, authored by Dr. Barry Sears. In the CrossFit Level 1 training handbook (which can be downloaded in its entirety at CrossFit.com), the nutrition and diet section of the course is essentially a condensed guide for the Zone Diet, an official declaration anchored in studies that have indicated how much diet affects our hormonal response to food, which in turn affects health. Sears has long believed that what you eat and how much you eat both have a critical effect on body chemistry. If you eat the wrong things and/or the wrong amounts of things over a significant period of time, you'll wear out the insulin system, get sick, and open the door for potentially fatal maladies like diabetes, heart disease, and cancer.

Sears makes the case for a balanced diet that avoids processed foods. He also suggests that the notion that weight loss is all about calories is flawed. Instead, weight control, overall health, and high-octane athletic performance all relate to the master hormone, insulin, and how the foods you eat trigger insulin production. High-carbohydrate diets—in particular ones fueled by pasta, grains, and packaged foods—tap the insulin response so frequently that we can become insulin-resistant on the cellular level, he says, which is the first step toward obesity and Type 2 adult-onset diabetes. They can also open the floodgate for other chronic diseases.

Sears recommends dialing down carbohydrate intake to somewhere in the neighborhood of 40 percent of your calories, with the remaining 60 percent of the calories in your diet split between fat and protein. In his lectures and books, he talks about how high-carb diets can burn out the receptors of the cells in your body that receive insulin. This produces a state called "hyperinsulinemia"—which essentially is insulin resistance, which basically means that you are prediabetic. Within the cells of someone who has reached this point, a chronic state of inflammation exists. A balanced diet, Sears says, can neutralize that person's hormonal response to food and provide an anti-inflammatory stabilization.

THE COMBINATION OF A HIGH-PERFORMANCE DIET AND CROSSFIT TRAINING CAN MOVE YOU INTO THE "JET STREAM OF ADAPTATION."

Hyperinsulinemia showed up for me in a blood test that was taken before I started working out at CrossFit Elysium. As a distance runner, I didn't expect to test positive. I later learned that hyperinsulinemia is not uncommon in runners. In a phone discussion, Dr. John Ivy, a leading researcher in sports nutrition at the University of Texas, explained how this happens. Studies have shown, he said, that older runners are able to keep a lurking blood-sugar problem like mine at bay—as long as they keep running. "When the subjects [of the studies] stopped running, within a week they were showing signs of developing diabetes," Dr. Ivy told me. This was possibly the case for me. I was injured and not running at the time of the blood test, and my diet was probably in the realm of 70 percent carbs, 10 percent protein, and 20 percent fat.

Sears started talking about all of this in the 1990s—stating that high-carb diets are killing Americans—and his view has slowly gained traction. Medical researchers began to take notice, producing their own studies with findings corroborating Sears's view. In a feature written for the *New York Times Magazine* in April 2011, nutrition journalist Gary Taubes profiled Robert Lustig from the School of Medicine at the University of California, San Francisco. Lustig is a pediatrician and an expert in childhood obesity who specializes in hormone disorders. His focus has been on the way sugar—in particular high-fructose corn syrup—has increased in the American diet. Sugar has become such a massive staple that, on average, every American consumes about 130 pounds of sugar per year, according to the U.S. Department of Agriculture. Lustig argues that sugar is a poison.

"If Lustig is right," Taubes wrote, "then our excessive consumption of sugar is the primary reason that the numbers of obese and diabetic Americans have skyrocketed in the past 30 years. But his argument implies more than that. If Lustig is right, it would mean that sugar is also the likely dietary cause of several other chronic ailments widely considered to be diseases of Western lifestyles: heart disease, hypertension and many common cancers among them."

CrossFit combines paleo thinking with the Zone. It looks at the percentage of carbs, the overall quantity of food, and the proportions of macronutrients you get in each meal. Eating a strict paleo diet, and supplanting carbs like pasta, bread, and cookies with carbs like spinach, tomatoes, and apples, say dedicated CrossFitters, will almost assuredly bring about improvements in health and workout performance. A reduction in carbohydrate intake, from 70 percent of an individual's calories to something much lower, occurs largely because of the caloric density of the foods involved in the switch to paleo eating. There are 220 calories in a cup of cooked pasta, whereas a cup of spinach has 7, a cup of cauliflower 25, and a medium apple 95. The paleo carbs also have much more fiber.

AVOIDING THE CRASH

At a CrossFit Level 1 training seminar, attendees hear a filtered-down description of the whys behind the macronutrient hows. Eat carbohydrates, and blood sugar rises; hence, insulin is released from the pancreas to store the excess sugar. Conversely, eat protein, and the hormone glucagon is released, which releases energy from the cells. Relative to carbohydrate and protein, fat is neutral in terms of a hormonal effect, but it does send a signal to the brain with a message. It says, "We're full," which prevents overeating.

Being in this neutralized state, what Sears calls "The Zone" is said to place the practitioner in a slipstream of energy. If you eat a Zone-balanced meal, it will leave you feeling energized and refreshed, whereas a massive bowl of pasta will have you wanting to crash underneath your desk at work.

At the CrossFit seminar, future coaches are taught that 40-30-30 (representing the percentages of carbs, protein, and fat, respectively) is a starting point. Every CrossFit athlete must accordingly pay attention to what is going on in the crashed-beneath-the-desk scenario. How you feel after you eat is the information you need to make whatever adjustments you need to make. According to the ideology of the Zone Diet, you're doing something wrong if you feel excessively tired or are still hungry after a meal. The goal is to feel satiated and energized for at least three hours, at which time you can bolster your state with another macronutrient-calibrated meal or snack.

Glassman says that, from what he's seen, the top CrossFit athletes take this calibration with the seriousness of a chemist. "You have to eat [meat and vegetables] and you have to get a scale and a measuring cup and you need accuracy and precision in your consumption or you'll never get in that jet stream of elite performance," he says. "You want top fuel performance, you need top fuel. You can't just piss into the gas tank. No one has ever demonstrated to me but inferior capacity on a diet where they didn't weigh and measure."

He adds, with characteristic aplomb, "On some level, I don't give a fuck. I'll go out with you right now and we can eat banana splits and drink beer all day. If you think you're going to get somewhere in terms of performance with this shit diet, though, I'll tell you you're high on crack. No one has ever done it. Take any cohort of people and get one of them to weigh and measure. And that one will pull away."

NUTRITION: THE MISSING PIECE

From the CrossFit point of view, nutrition is vital. Metaphors for nutrition abound in lectures and training sessions. As mentioned above, it is seen as the foundation of the CrossFit pyramid, the basis for health and wellness. For Glassman, it is one of the two oars necessary to propel the CrossFit boat; without it, you're going in circles. For others, it turns out to be the missing piece of a puzzle.

Nicole Carroll, co-director of training at CrossFit HQ, would likely agree with all of these views. One of Carroll's lectures on nutrition is archived in the *CrossFit Journal*'s "Classics" category. She has also written articles for the journal on nutrition (including one entitled "Get Off the Crack," her personal story of conquering a sugar addiction). In the "Classics" video, Carroll brings up the correlation between nutrition and high performance: "As trainers, we often see someone come that is hitting the workouts consistently, with a good amount of intensity, and they make gains, they make gains and then they plateau or even regress. We call this a failure to thrive. This is a nutrition-related issue. If you're working out without eating right, you will not get the results. You'll get half the results. You will not survive and definitely not thrive in this program unless you're eating right."

Briana Drost, the dispatcher, certainly found these words to be true. In January 2011, feeling more fit from her training but still seeking body-shape changes, Drost began to focus on her diet. She was shocked when, in the course of four weeks, 15 pounds seemed to melt away from her body. It was, indeed, the missing piece.

Chang says that Elysium intentionally refrains from pushing members on diet. But when someone like Drost gets frustrated with the rate of improvement, they will advise a dietary remake. "The reason Briana's progress sped up so much when she paid attention to her diet is twofold," Chang says. "For one, the human body is like a machine, and any machine is dependent on quality fuel to run optimally. Put garbage for fuel in, and you get garbage out. In practical terms what that means is feeling lethargic throughout the day, sleeping poorly, and performing suboptimally in workouts."

Eating right enabled Briana "to train harder, recover better, and have more energy to make it into the gym more often," he adds. And, "under those conditions, it's easy to see why her progress would improve." The second reason her progress improved was that she "started giving her body macronutrients in the quantities it needed. Under these circumstances, it's actually difficult for an overweight person to *not* lose weight." In other words, quality and quantity were the keys.

The application of a Zone-paleo approach to food requires planning. In Drost's case, it required preparing and packing up enough meals and snacks to get her through a 12-hour workshift, then school, then intern assignments as a counselor, and then her workout. No one said that eating right was easy, especially at first. But the payoff was rapid.

Estrada remembers Drost's January acceleration. "I won't comment on anyone's weight loss unless it's a big change, one I'm sure of," he says. "There was a day when I saw a woman in a hallway. Her back was to me and I didn't know who it was. She turned around and it was Briana. I had to do a double-take—she had completely transformed." After that six-month mark, Drost startled coworkers as well, who asked her the same question she'd asked months before. "They said, 'Holy shit! What have you been doing?'"

After watching Drost's consistency and commitment to the program, Chang was not surprised by the progress. "Briana is a very strong-willed and dedicated person," he says. "She is willing to work hard and make sacrifices to get what she wants—in this case, physical fitness. In this day and age, those are particularly remarkable traits."

Chang notes that "most people talk about what they want but are completely unwilling to lift a finger to help themselves get there. It's as if they expect the world to do them a favor. Quite honestly, I think this is infuriating. By contrast, for financial reasons, Briana had to decide between cable TV and training with us—and she canceled her TV subscription. I bet 99 percent of couch potatoes out there would have prioritized things the other way, thereby generating a convenient excuse why they 'couldn't work out.'" He adds, "Her job involves her working long nights, and often she'll train *after* having been up all night. She is that dedicated."

As a result of adding the nutrition piece of the puzzle and continuing to work hard in training, "Briana deserves all of the success she's had, because she's earned it," says Chang. "Briana really is an example of the phenomenon of 'success breeding success.' Each achievement she's made, each milestone she's passed, has only served to drive her to new heights. It's amazing to watch as a coach and a friend."

> EATING RIGHT ENABLED BRIANA "TO TRAIN HARDER, RECOVER BETTER, AND HAVE MORE ENERGY TO MAKE IT INTO THE GYM MORE OFTEN. UNDER THOSE CONDITIONS, IT'S EASY TO SEE WHY HER PROGRESS WOULD IMPROVE."

A CRITICAL LOOK AT CONVENTIONAL NUTRITION

Chang is an intense, no-bullshit character who speaks freely and passionately on the subjects to which he devotes himself. He also suffers no fools. Once he made a casual reference to a poker night he hosted at his house, and I casually expressed interest in dropping in, assuming it was a casual game. He promptly said that he'd loan me some books on the subject of poker—and I realized his poker nights were not as casual as I'd imagined. Later, I found out that Chang actually helped pay his way through medical school by hitting poker tables in casinos. Not only that, his skill at poker helped him and his wife, Alessandra Wall, buy their first house. I never did make it to his poker night, and I'd bet that my personal savings account is all the better for it.

Chang brings the same intensity and devotion that he brings to poker to the gym. You can see quickly that he has little tolerance for anyone trying to get something for nothing, and he has kicked people out of the gym whom he has perceived as having attitude problems, even when the gym was brand new and just building its membership base.

Chang offers a one-on-one coaching service for gym members who want to chase specific goals, but he has the following prerequisite:

MOTIVATED PEOPLE ONLY

By entering here, you agree to give 100% of what you have. There are no excuses or second chances. Every day, every moment is an opportunity to excel, to be more, to achieve your best. Do not squander your time going through the motions. Train hard and get results. At the end of the day, look in the mirror and ask yourself if you gave your all. If you don't have that level of commitment, don't waste your time or ours.

This intense level of commitment is what Chang expects his athletes to give in exchange for results. And Chang's dedication to them is also extreme. In considering this level of dedication, I found myself wondering how long such complete discipline was sustainable.

As it turns out, even Chang does have at least one weakness when it comes to nutrition: coffee. I glimpsed this human side during a talk on nutrition, when he was asked about how coffee figures into the big picture. Should we look into leaving it behind? The question came from the front row. Chang took a deep pull from a large Peet's coffee cup.

"Look," he said. "I am a caffeine addict. But on the grand scale of things, the effect of coffee is null. What you want to focus on is getting rid of sugar and eating real food. Coffee has a relatively insignificant impact."

The significant impacts, he says, come from agribusiness. What gets Chang really fired up is his fervent belief that agribusiness has the American political system "by the balls," and the result is that agribusiness is guiding the conversation about nutrition.

"I'd say the biggest flaw with the U.S. health-care system is that the current conception of what constitutes healthy versus unhealthy eating is completely wrong," Chang told me when I asked him his take on the subject. "Everything is based off the food pyramid, which was created by the USDA."

Chang believes the backstory is political in nature. "It was flawed science funded by the agricultural mega-industries, like the corn and grain industries, coupled with a political agenda to demonize; this is what . . . created the food pyramid as we know it today."

Chang's stance is essentially the same as that of the rest of the CrossFit community and Barry Sears: "The high-carb/low-fat diet all of us have been taught to eat is probably the single biggest killer in the Western world today. It is directly responsible for diabetes, hypertension, obesity, and heart disease." Hospitals are filled with people who tried to follow the USDA food pyramid, he says.

The bottom line is that "cardiovascular disease has been the number one cause of death in America for decades now, and diabetes, hypertension, obesity, [and] CV disease are all interrelated—if you have one, you probably have another, and each in turn can result from another":

All of us who have "seen the light" are facing a monumental uphill battle. The amount of misinformation out there is staggering. Many people, both the layperson and MD alike, hate to have their long-held beliefs challenged. This means that getting people to understand what they've been taught is wrong and to change what they're doing is almost impossible. Lastly, the mega-corporations that control the grain and corn industries have a vested interest in keeping things the way they are. These are multibillion-dollar industries, and in politics, money talks. It's no wonder that there's little to no political will to change how Americans eat.

Chang sees the situation changing very slowly over the coming generations. "People, little by little, will start to see the light and vote with their pocketbooks. In this sense, CrossFit can contribute on the grassroots level simply by opening some people's eyes."

Although, if this is true, people had better start voting with their pocketbooks more frequently. As has been well documented in many sources in recent years, Type 2 diabetes is increasing in children. This is a new development—in the past, Type 2 diabetes was also called "adult-onset diabetes" because it was so rare in children. Today, it is more and more common, with obesity among children being considered a major risk factor. And, to make matters worse, the drugs typically administered for adults with Type 2 diabetes are not always effective for young patients. These children face the very real risk of going blind, having their limbs amputated, and ending up with chronic diseases such as heart disease and cancer.

It's time to take a closer look at paleolithic eating and the Zone Diet, not just for CrossFitters, but for anyone currently eating a carb-rich, sugar-loaded diet.

THE NUTRITION CHALLENGE

The primary educational tool for nutrition at CrossFit affiliates is a "challenge." At CrossFit Elysium, in August 2011, I entered my first Nutrition Challenge, excited about the game of it, but admittedly a bit nervous at the prospect of overhauling my nutrition on such a large scale.

The challenge, a six-week deal, started on a Monday and worked on a point system. You were awarded points (or docked points) for what you ate for each meal. Eating an all-paleo meal would get you 1 point; a Zoned meal would get you 2 points; and a Zone-paleo meal, meaning all paleo-friendly foods, but weighed and measured to Zone proportions, would get you 3 points. If all the carbs came strictly from vegetables (and not vegetables and fruits), you could get a bonus point. Points were awarded for training, too—so many points for doing three CrossFit workouts per week, a bonus if you got to Elysium four times per week, and a max bonus if you made it five times per week. Additional points were won or lost based on how much sleep you got, how much water you drank, and whether you took fish oil supplements every day.

On day one, everyone was weighed, had their body fat measured, and did a CrossFit benchmark workout called "Cindy." Cindy is a CrossFit AMRAP. It includes the following:

CINDY
20-minute AMRAP
5 pull-ups, 10 push-ups, 15 air squats

On August 22, I performed Cindy. As best as I could, since I had just learned how to do them, I employed kipping pull-ups, then the push-ups and air squats, wincing through a first set. I ended up doing 11 rounds in the 20 minutes, and when I finished, I sprawled out in my own sweat, flat on the floor, wondering how it could be possible to do any more than I had just done. I had done the workout

"RX," or as prescribed, meaning that I didn't scale any of the movements with modifications. From that moment on, the challenge actually started for me—for six weeks, what I ate mattered, and my retest of Cindy down the road would be the moment of truth for how much it mattered.

A large poster at CrossFit Elysium would announce our progress week by week. Everyone competing in the challenge was listed along with the initial body-fat measurements, weights, and Cindy times. Six columns had been drawn out for our subsequent weekly scores. In typical CrossFit style, everyone would know what everyone else was doing.

I bought a small digital scale and a measuring cup, which was for portion size. According to both Sears and Glassman, it's not about weighing and measuring your food for the rest of your life. Rather, they say, this is something you have to do just at first, so you can get an idea of how much you're eating. Measuring your food also gives you a feel for eyeballing the correct proportions of protein to carbs to fat at a single meal.

Through the Sears calculator, I figured out how much protein I would need per day: 120 grams. These grams were to be divided over the course of three meals and two snacks. Within each meal, I would also add carbohydrates and fats in the correct ratios.

"It's hard to do," Dr. Sears told me in an interview, "especially with paleo-type foods. What I try to do in my books is make it as simple as possible." (In his books, Sears does a nice job of making the techniques of the diet clear and accessible. When I first had the diet explained to me, I suffered brain-lock over how macronutrient intake was coordinated into "blocks," but Sears writes with a very clear, teacherly style, and I grasped it quickly.)

That said, the first week was pretty rough. I had purchased several of Sears's books in the hope that I would use the recipes. The protein part was easy. Four or five ounces of chicken, fish, or red meat are pretty easy to weigh and cook. The fat part was easy, too. Teaspoons of olive oil, tablespoons of avocado, or a rather sadly low number of nuts (for a snack you might be allowed one macadamia nut, for example) may not sound like much, but at least this part is easy to follow. That's all the fat you get. Nuts do not come by the handful, as I had always practiced.

The carbs were the tough part, in two respects. Calculating the number of carbs from an assortment of vegetables was somewhat tricky. At first I shuttled back and forth between an online calorie calculator and whatever vegetable I had chopped up on the cutting board. Cauliflower, cabbage, kale, spinach, radishes, onions, you name it. The more components, the more I felt like I was working on an advanced math degree.

This is when I discovered a newfound love for bags of frozen vegetables. Already measured, cut, and mixed up, they saved me a lot of trouble. And they made it possible, even easy, to get all my carb calories from vegetables, thereby allowing me to gain the coveted points.

The second problem, though, still lay in trying to earn that one last extra point for a Zone-paleo meal that I could only get if I obtained all my carb calories from vegetables. Unless you include a vegetable like sweet potatoes, you might be talking about a small mountain range of vegetables to get your quota. If I had 28 grams of protein in my dinner, I would need 36 grams of carbohydrate for the correct Zone proportions. One night, I got all my carbs for a meal like this from asparagus. One spear of asparagus has 2.5 grams of carbohydrate. So that's 14.5 spears of asparagus I had to eat. I continued eating asparagus long after I was full and was tired of asparagus, but I did get that last point.

> EVENTUALLY, I ACQUIRED NEW ROUTINES. I NOT ONLY BEGAN COOKING MY DINNERS IN NEW WAYS BUT ALSO STARTED PACKING A LUNCH AND SNACKS IN THE EVENING, PREPARING THEM AHEAD OF TIME AND PUTTING THEM INTO TUPPERWARE CONTAINERS TO GRAB AND TAKE THE NEXT DAY.

For breakfast, I usually had egg whites along with one whole egg and virtual truckloads of spinach. Other days, I just went for the Zone-only points and made a blender drink from a recipe I found in a *CrossFit Journal* article on nutrition. It called for milk, frozen strawberries and blueberries, protein powder, and a "scoop" of cashews. I only got 2 points for the meal, but it was all I could manage on those mornings. As Sears said in my interview with him, the tough part of doing the Zone-paleo diet is really twofold: It's a matter of time and accessibility, both of which can be problematic on busy days when you are away from home for hours. I ended up eating a lot of the same things over and over again.

The good news is that it did get easier. Eventually, I acquired new routines. I not only began cooking my dinners in new ways but also started packing a lunch and snacks in the evening, preparing them ahead of time and putting them into Tupperware containers to grab and take the next day.

For lunches and dinners, I had many meals that were cooked up from frozen vegetables, with chicken or turkey for protein and an avocado for the fat. Snacks often consisted of an ounce of chicken with a complement of fruits, vegetables, and nuts, measured out to Zone proportions. Some nights I had a final snack of a 4-ounce glass of red wine and an ounce of chicken.

Travel made things a bit difficult at times, and my weekly point totals sagged here and there, but there was no mistaking that my overall diet was much altered from before the start of the Nutrition Challenge.

When the results came six weeks later, they were impressive. My body-fat percentage dropped 2 percentage points, from 17 percent to 15 percent. We retested the Cindy met-con, and instead of doing 11 rounds, I did 14 rounds. I had gained exactly three full rounds, meaning that I had performed an additional 15 pull-ups, an additional 30 push-ups, and an additional 45 air squats. Considering how flattened I was by the first test, I would have been happily surprised with a one-round gain. Three sort of stunned me.

Most critically, I had my blood retested after the challenge for signs of hyperinsulinemia. The high-blood-sugar levels had been cut in half, and I was offi-cially in the safe zone. (Although I still had room for improvement—according to Dr. Sears, getting levels of cellular inflammation to rock-bottom levels is the way to prepare your body for top athletic performance.)

I was convinced. This was working. I had to finally let go of my lengthy con-viction that as long as I was running I could afford to eat whatever I wanted. Sad, but ridiculously true.

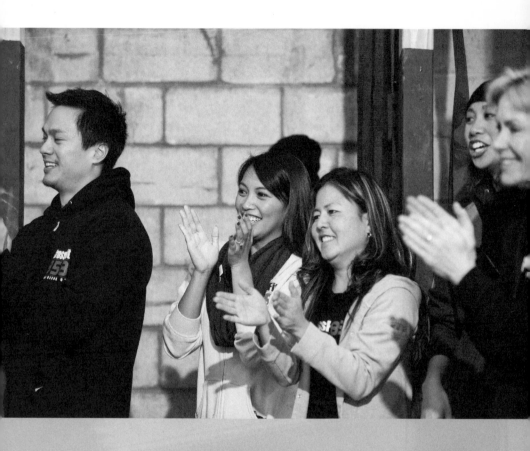

CULTFIT

6

THE COMMUNITY AND SOCIOLOGY
OF CROSSFIT

ONCE AFTER A WORKOUT AT ELYSIUM, CROSSFITTER DAVE BENNETT AND I WERE chatting outside the main workout area, near the gym entrance, about a one-day competition he had watched in Orange County. We stopped our conversation for a moment as a member, a woman dressed for training, came in with her baby daughter in a stroller. Checking out the day's workout, she noticed that it included sprints outside the building. She asked if anyone could keep an eye on her baby during that part of the workout. Before Dave or I could reply, a chorus of assents rang out from around the box, with everyone within earshot volunteering to watch the little girl.

Dave looked over at me and smiled. "I don't have any kids yet, but I'll tell you, if I did, I'd leave my kid with anyone in here, any day."

The implication was clear: The sense of community here was strong. There was a great amount of trust among the people at the gym. Some members were newer than others and consequently didn't know everyone as well, but this didn't seem to matter. CrossFit Elysium had established a community, and everyone had each other's backs.

This brand of community likely varies from gym to gym. On the day Dave said this to me, there were approximately 80 members total at Elysium, a small, tight-knit group. I wondered whether the same dynamic existed on a larger level. Would the same camaraderie be apparent at CrossFit events? I would soon have many chances to find out.

When I went to Carson, California, just south of Los Angeles for the 2011 Reebok CrossFit Games, I ran into an acquaintance one afternoon at the Home Depot Center Sports Complex where the Games were held. I'd worked out with him two weeks prior, at CrossFit Southie, when I was visiting Boston. It was a surprise to run into him, since the last time I'd seen him we were on the East Coast, more than 3,000 miles away. We started talking about the spectacle of the Games and the mass gathering of CrossFitters from around the country and the world.

"Have you noticed how people are here?" he asked.

"How do you mean?"

"Everyone is so nice to one another. All these crowded situations, lines at the concession stands, in the parking lot, everything. They're so considerate. You're walking into the bathroom, and people don't run you over on their way out. They smile and let you through. People are smiling and out to do whatever they can to help you out."

It was true. In contrast to what you might expect from people awash with tattoos and a sort of AC/DC-meets-gymnastics fashion sense, such as bobby socks and radiantly colored minimalist footwear, the throngs of CrossFitters in attendance were extraordinarily polite and helpful to one another.

Maybe this is why people from outside CrossFit looking in—as I once was—conclude that CrossFit must be some sort of eccentric, masochistic fitness cult. Even CrossFitters acknowledge that a cultish reputation has developed. In online forums and social-networking threads, the phrase "drinking the Kool-Aid" surfaces frequently, albeit in tongue-in-cheek fashion. The reference of course is to the mindless followers who drank poisoned juice in the 1978 Jonestown Massacre. But there is no conventional brainwashing in CrossFit, no selling of flowers at the airport or worshipping of sociopathic gurus; indeed, CrossFit isn't a cult by any standard definition. But a question does come to mind when you see members of the close-knit community interact. The social structures typical at CrossFit gyms resemble in some ways those of another, more well-established institution in society. If it's not a cult, then that question must be asked: Is CrossFit a church?

IS CROSSFIT A CHURCH?

According to Dr. Allison Belger, a psychologist who co-owns four affiliate gyms with her husband, TJ Belger, and is the author of *The Power of Community: CrossFit and the Force of Human Connection*, the answer is yes, if you subtract the religious dimension. "If we are open to the idea of being in a community where people may look different, come from different backgrounds, and have different interests, as it tends to happen in a CrossFit community, then there's the possibility that a CrossFit affiliate can offer a similar function that a church does," Belger told me in a discussion over her book. She adds, "That's one of the missions of religion—to let go of all of the differences and unite a group within a common purpose."

In 2008, Belger witnessed the emergence of a CrossFit community when her husband, TJ, converted his personal training gym into a CrossFit box. Belger noticed it wasn't for everyone, she told me, implying that the nature of CrossFit—the high-intensity exercise and the heavy emphasis on the group dynamic—was such that a certain percentage of people trying it couldn't get out of the gym fast enough. "Some will say, 'I can't stand this. Get me the F out of here.'" But it was apparent that for others, the structure of CrossFit was exactly what they needed, not only in order to find success in their fitness goals but also in order to fill the social fissures that occur so often in the era of Facebook. They embraced the group support, the kind of attention they received when being coached, and the overall goal-setting and recordkeeping methods used in CrossFit. The powerful community aspect of CrossFit, says Belger, was clearly an important ancillary benefit of working out in a CrossFit gym. People met who might not ever have crossed paths otherwise, and they became friends. "CrossFit fosters and facilitates the breaking down of barriers."

> "CROSSFIT FOSTERS AND FACILITATES THE BREAKING DOWN OF BARRIERS."

The poignant moment for Belger in terms of how a CrossFit community can transcend the boundaries of an ordinary gym came when Margie Simenstad, who had been a member of the Belgers' gym for six months, was told the tragic news that her brother, Joe, had fallen two stories from an apartment building in New York City. He had sustained traumatic brain and bodily injuries, and, to be with him, Simenstad had boarded a red-eye flight for New York.

As reported in *The Power of Community*, Simenstad, sitting alone on the plane, reached out to the gym community in a way she never before had imagined. "I was doing my best to think positive thoughts about Joe, but I felt so small and insubstantial—that there was nothing I could do on my own to help Joe," she later reported. "I am an extremely practical person who finds it extremely hard to stomach anything remotely resembling touchy-feely new-age beliefs. But dire circumstances can cause you to depart from the norm."

Simenstad reasoned that the possibility of a larger number of people thinking positive thoughts for her brother could help. She sent a text message to TJ, explaining the situation, and asked if he could relay a request to the gym community: Please send your positive thoughts toward my brother.

TJ Belger published a post on Simenstad's situation on the affiliate blog along with her unusual request. For the next week, Simenstad received an outpouring of e-mails and phone calls "from people I knew casually or not at all [sending] the most caring and concerned messages to me, with people offering their support, good thoughts, help with my kids and kind words.... The idea that so many people were at home holding Joe in their thoughts kept me going through some very dark moments. . . . I realized quite clearly and profoundly how lucky I was to have joined the community at TJ's Gym."

ALONE IN A CROWD

It doesn't take much research to see evidence of one of the primary worries of psychologists and sociologists in the Facebook era—that technology will further erode the sense of community in America.

In his 1995 essay "Bowling Alone: America's Declining Social Capital," published in the *Journal of Democracy* (later revised and published as a book under the title *Bowling Alone: The Collapse and Revival of American Community*, in 2000), Robert Putnam argued that both community and direct, face-to-face contact had been declining since 1950. The title of the essay was a reference to the finding that, by 1995, the number of people who were bowling in leagues had shrunk, despite the fact that more Americans were bowling overall. The research suggested that this was an example of how Americans were isolating themselves and rejecting contact with civic groups and other types of social clubs.

Consider that in 1995, when the essay first came out, dial-up modems and e-mail were just catching on. Social networking and texting were years away. Smartphone apps, with their addictive way of keeping us completely absorbed and unaware of much of our surroundings, were not even on the horizon. For Putnam, television and suburban life were largely to blame. His theories have proven more and more prescient as technology has advanced.

Recent reporting has discussed the impact of social networking as a substitute for actually being with people. In *The Atlantic*, in an article entitled "Is Facebook Making Us Lonely?" published in May 2012, author Stephen Marche reported on the public-health ramifications of a "loneliness" epidemic:

A 2010 AARP survey found that 35 percent of adults older than 45 were chronically lonely, as opposed to 20 percent of a similar group only a decade earlier. According to a major study by a leading scholar of the subject, roughly 20 percent of Americans—about 60 million people—are unhappy with their lives because of loneliness. Across the Western world, physicians and nurses have begun to speak openly of an epidemic of loneliness.

. . .

... Being lonely is extremely bad for your health. If you're lonely, you're more likely to be put in a geriatric home at an earlier age than a similar person who isn't lonely. You're less likely to exercise. You're more likely to be obese. You're less likely to survive a serious operation and more likely to have hormonal imbalances. You are at greater risk of inflammation. Your memory may be worse. You are more likely to be depressed, to sleep badly, and to suffer dementia and general cognitive decline.

Sherry Turkle is a psychologist and professor at the Massachusetts Institute of Technology and author of the book *Alone Together: Why We Expect More from Technology and Less from Each Other* (2011). Turkle is frank in her analysis of what she perceives as modern technology's tendency to allow people to avoid the emotional drain of face-to-face conversations as well as the dangers this may entail. She points to the advent of artificial intelligence devices, such as the Siri iPhone application. More than a practical tool, these technological inventions seem to provide people with a virtual friend to talk to. In one experiment she conducted, a robotic baby seal was given to an older woman in a senior care facility. The robot was designed to appear to look into her eyes as if it were listening. Turkle reported that the woman began talking to the seal about the loss of her child.

Others have used the robotic seal, which was developed by Takanori Shibata at the National Institute of Advanced Industrial Science and Technology in Japan, to ease the loneliness of patients with dementia. But loneliness is not a malady confined to the elderly, and the idea of finding comfort in talking to a robotic seal seems like something out of a sci-fi horror novel. Nevertheless, it may offer insight into why those who have found a CrossFit community are often so enthusiastic about it. In making an argument for bringing real conversations with real people back into our lives, Turkle wrote, in a *New York Times* op-ed piece in April 2012:

We've become accustomed to a new way of being "alone together." Technology-enabled, we are able to be with one another, and also elsewhere, connected to wherever we want to be. We want to customize our lives. We want to move in and out of where we are because the thing we value most is control over where we focus our attention. We have gotten used to the idea of being in a tribe of one, loyal to our own party.

. . .

We are tempted to think that our little "sips"of online connection add up to a big gulp of real conversation. But they don't. E-mail, Twitter, Facebook, all of these have their places—in politics, commerce, romance and friendship. But no matter how valuable, they do not substitute for conversation.

In a 2011 commencement speech delivered to Kenyon College, novelist Jonathan Franzen, a self-described "cranky 51-year-old," spoke of the temptations of hiding from others through the use of technology:

> To go through a life painlessly is to have not lived. Even just to say to yourself, "Oh, I'll get to that love and pain stuff later, maybe in my 30s," is to consign yourself to 10 years of merely taking up space on the planet and burning up its resources. Of being (and I mean this in the most damning sense of the word) a consumer.
>
> . . .
>
> When you stay in your room and rage or sneer or shrug your shoulders, as I did for many years, the world and its problems are impossibly daunting. But when you go out and put yourself in real relation to real people, or even just real animals, there's a very real danger that you might love some of them.

And who knows what might happen to you then?

In fact, CrossFit communities don't eschew computers, Facebook, or Twitter. They embrace them with passion. CrossFit Elysium's lively Facebook activity is a shining example of this. But to the points of Franzen and Turkle—and as demonstrated in the story of Marge Simenstad—the Internet communications are supplemental to the very real and apparently connective experience of suffering alongside one another through a daily workout.

FINDING COMMUNION

Belger's observation that a CrossFit box has a unique way of drawing in a diverse group of individuals and enabling them to form an unlikely community interested me because I had observed the principle in action at CrossFit Elysium. Discovering that sense of community was, for me, unexpected. San Diego is a commuter city. The people who live there spend an inordinate amount of time grinding through traffic on the interstates. I'd lived there for seven years, and, like many others, had no sense of local community apart from work.

When the CrossFit mantra—"Making the Uncomfortable Comfortable"—was first explained to me, I was on the edge of joining those whom Belger had observed running for the door. The slogan refers not just to the discomfort of working out but to the discomfort of meeting new people. Workouts inevitably begin with the coach making sure that everyone meets everyone else—but I was fresh out of a divorce and content to develop a bunker-like apartment that would allow me to keep new human contact to the barest minimum.

Once I became enchanted with the workouts, though, and started showing up regularly, I couldn't keep my fortress-like attitude going. One of the first things to win me over was the preternatural ability of the CrossFit Elysium coaches to memorize not only names, mine included, but also specific workout achievements linked with those names. Coach Paul Estrada was especially impressive in this regard. Although at the time Elysium had 80 members, I soon discovered that he could recall what I had lifted in workouts four or five weeks beforehand. He could teach a large group, including several new people, and almost instantly pick up and recall all of their names.

Since the coaches used names, it was only a matter of weeks before I was on a first-name basis with more than 10 of the Elysium members. And perhaps the nature of the workouts themselves tends to elicit camaraderie—the anxiety of facing one of your least favorite met-cons, the shared challenge of grinding your way through something tougher than you think you can handle. It is in such hardships that people develop a mutual respect and, as I discovered, a caring attitude about your compatriots. Elysium had parties and get-togethers, including a Halloween party, a Christmas party, and special WODs to honor the achievements of members. And beyond the gym Elysium used Facebook to continue the conversation—these web-based channels of communication thrived.

What this also fueled, of course, was a powerful mechanism to help people achieve fitness goals. Because constantly varied/anaerobic training yields such rapid results, fitness progress in CrossFit is exceptional compared with conventional routes, and though much of this is due to the nature of the workouts themselves, some of it is no doubt also due to the level of support, the friendly competition, and the sense of accountability and motivation that a community fosters. People showed up consistently, people worked hard consistently, and people addressed ancillary paths like nutrition and stretching to enhance their progress.

THE KEY INGREDIENTS

In December 2001, Greg Amundson started training at Glassman's original CrossFit gym. Amundson thus witnessed the emergence of the first vital CrossFit community, which became a template for the thousands of affiliates that exist today. It became clear to Amundson that the bonding agent of the community was how much effort the work involved.

"We concentrated on the process as opposed to the results, and in CrossFit, quality of effort is the process," Amundson told me. "The gym was a magic place. Your status outside the gym meant nothing. Whatever problems you may have had at work or in your relationships, you left that at the door. We'd have the '3, 2, 1, go,' and all of that was gone." The culture in the gym, he says, was such that you received respect and accolades not by whether you were the best in the gym, or the second best, or even the next to last. What was rewarded was how hard you tried.

"The WOD was a great equalizer," Amundson says. "The WOD didn't care whether you had a college degree or whether you just got a promotion at work, or if you came in first. The only thing that mattered was the effort you gave that day, at that workout."

Amundson adds that it is the very difficulty of the workout that brings out the best in people: "In the gym, doing the WOD, you have an honest-to-goodness fight on your hands. After you've fought your way through it, you know you accomplished something. You're sweating. Your throat is burning. You have calluses. You know you did something hard, something real."

In April 2011, I went to hear Belger give a talk to a group of urban community designers who were interested in the relationship between habitats and groups of people. She summarized her perspective on the necessary framework to make a community successful. It wasn't what you might expect. "To make a community really work," she said, "you need to have some suffering involved. It's got to be a little gritty. Think about the most difficult things you've ever done in your life and how often those things were accomplished because you were part of a group or a team."

A Special Forces officer, Captain Michael Perry, once called Greg Glassman and told him that CrossFit helped him identify what galvanized the kind of camaraderie necessary for an effective military team. "It's agony coupled with laughter," he told Glassman. CrossFitters push each other through a hard workout and then spend time cracking up with one another over it all.

"All great things within whatever province in every domain comes to those willing to suffer, endure sacrifice, and commit," Glassman said in CrossFit.com interview with Tony Budding, director of CrossFit Media. "This is true in business, it's true in physics or learning to play the violin. You can't get better without sacrifice. It requires a tolerance to discomfort. Getting fit is hard and frustrating. What all CrossFitters share in total is that all good things come from sacrifice and discomfort. It's a stoic sort of mindset."

The people who end up doing CrossFit, Glassman believes, "don't believe you can get something for nothing." The ones who think there's an easy path and don't like to suffer, in other words, are filtered out of the gyms. "Once you get rid of the people who want something for nothing, you're co-selecting a whole bunch of admirable traits. Thieves disappear."

"TO MAKE A COMMUNITY REALLY WORK, YOU NEED TO HAVE SOME SUFFERING INVOLVED. IT'S GOT TO BE A LITTLE GRITTY."

"Belief in your own potential is hugely uniting," Glassman continued. "I don't care who or what you are. If you believe that we can enjoy one another's company, support each other toward achieving some physical goals, that we'll mutually support one another in something that happens here collaboratively, in what is a positive experience in a collaborative way, then you'll come to see you're one of us."

In addition to a strong sense of identity with a community, Glassman's most recent initiatives are similar to another essential characteristic of a church: doing good works for others. The following are some of the additions that Glassman hopes affiliates pick up within their own businesses: offering SAT preparation programs; actively working on clean-water projects in Kenya; providing financial support for an Infant Swimming Resource and a program to address the startling statistics in regard to death and brain damage suffered through child drowning incidents; and ongoing support of soldiers, police, and firefighters.

One particular story that personified the community dynamic of CrossFit in a way that I could relate to was the story of 37-year-old Meghan Kearney, now a social worker in San Francisco who helps troubled teenagers get their lives on track. She's also a core member of San Francisco CrossFit, something that five years ago, she told me, she never would have remotely imagined or considered doing. Things started to change in 2007, when Kearney, then living in Colorado, was diagnosed with breast cancer. It was during the weeks of chemotherapy that she and her boyfriend broke up, intensifying the trauma of fighting cancer. The fight against cancer would include surgery, reconstruction, and hair loss. She decided to leave Colorado and go to San Francisco, where she moved in with a lifelong friend, Gretchen Weber.

"I didn't have a job and didn't know that many people in the city,"she recalls. "I spent most of my time staring out the window." Weber had been one of the first members of SFCF and eventually coaxed Kearney into coming to the gym. Over breakfast, talking about that period of time in her life, Kearney remembers few of the details, but one especially powerful image remained. She recalled a day that she was being coached to do a pull-up. She was still regrowing the hair she had lost during the chemotherapy treatments; the cancer treatment had also devoured her lean muscle tissue. But her strength was slowly resurfacing.

"I was circled by everyone in the gym—the coaches, the other athletes, every-one telling me I could do it," she said. And Kearney did it—the first pull-up of her life. "San Francisco CrossFit is what helped me get a foothold on my life."

In retracing my own steps, I recall the first time I foraged through the CrossFit.com website. My awe at the images of athleticism was counterbal-anced by an aversion for some of the more extreme examples of what sometimes accompanies unhinged enthusiasm for CrossFit. Peeling off strips of skin from the hands (a common problem in conjunction with overuse of barbells, pull-up bars, and gymnastics rings) and postworkout vomiting are seen by some as badges of honor. For me it was a red flag. How stupid is it to desire ripping flesh off your hands? Or throwing up your lunch? (I would later realize I was in the majority on this one. The coaches I've met generally try to steer their athletes away from such conditions.) But I couldn't get over how fit the CrossFitter athletes were. They had an almost elastic quality to the way they moved.

Though I wasn't dealing with anything close to the challenges Kearney had faced with cancer, I was most certainly in a dark place with no plan or structure to prevent me from tunneling deeper. And at the time, I was not looking for a community. The idea of meeting new people would have been about as attrac-tive to me as having my fingernails ripped out and then washing dishes with gasoline. But I didn't yet know about the CrossFit community. I had no idea that CrossFit had ritualized making sure you got to know everyone—until it was too late and I was already getting to know them. And by that point I realized that most CrossFitters weren't fitness crackpots, but down-to-earth people who made a point of being neighborly in a sincere, heartfelt way.

CrossFit offered me, as it did Kearney, a fixed rope during a time when I was most certainly sliding off of a cliff. I began to see the skepticism in the eyes of non-CrossFitters as I zealously encouraged them to try CrossFit. I didn't blame them. I had the evangelical vibe of the freshly converted.

When I ended my membership at CrossFit Elysium on the last day of February 2012, as I was preparing to move to San Francisco, it was a profoundly difficult experience. This was surprising, because I'd only been there six months. After my last workout at Elysium, a few of us sat together on benches and chatted. I was asked about my upcoming move. How I was getting there? What box would I join? I was struck with sadness, knowing I was leaving these people who had become so important to me in such a short time. The friendships had come as such a surprise, and yet now they felt so indispensable. I felt a remarkable loss in having to say good-bye.

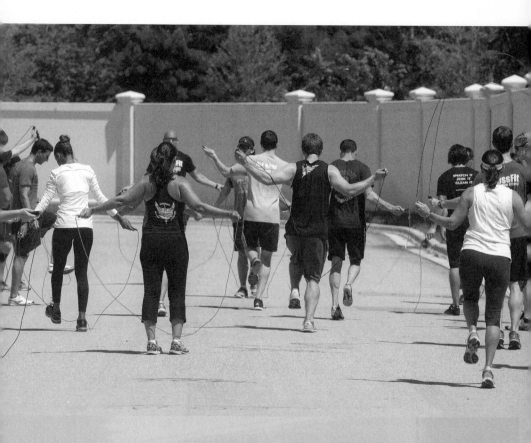

IRENE'S JOURNEY 7

A CASE STUDY

DROP INTO THE 4:30 P.M. CLASS AT CROSSFIT ELYSIUM, MONDAY THROUGH FRIDAY, and you'll be working out alongside Irene Mejia. Irene will introduce herself to you and welcome you to the gym. She may give you a hug after the workout, even though you'll both likely be soaked in sweat. Irene goes full tilt, sometimes emitting a war cry-like scream during her attempts at personal-record lifts. She's almost overly consistent in her training, going to CrossFit six times per week, a rate that I personally couldn't keep up without becoming overtrained. On weekends she adds to the count by visiting other CrossFit affiliates (as of June 2012 she has visited and worked out at 48 different gyms). She has a school-girl's smile and a twinkle in her eye that is warm and puts you in a good mood. She's Hispanic, loves Disneyland, and loves salsa dancing. She lives life like a basketball player in a full court press.

One other thing about Irene Mejia: When she joined CrossFit Elysium in June 2010, she could barely handle the two blocks of walking required to get from her home to the gym. She weighed 415 pounds and was suffering from morbid obesity.

Irene is 38 years old. But whether it's childhood obesity, adolescent obesity, or adult obesity, it seems like every talk show, news show, blog, and online or print news source has repeatedly told what seems to be the health-news story of the decade. And the story is true. Obesity has become a major and troubling problem.

According to the Centers for Disease Control and Prevention, more than one-third of the adults in the United States are obese. The CDC reports that the "medical costs associated with obesity were estimated at $147 billion" in 2008, and the medical costs paid by insurance companies for obese individuals were much higher than those for individuals of normal weight ($1,429 higher, on average, to be exact).

Obesity is a major risk factor for diabetes in adults and children. It can also lead to hypertension, respiratory ailments, and other problems, including heart disease and cancer.

Any fitness program worth its salt needs to address this obesity epidemic. So what does CrossFit have to offer by way of a solution to a problem that is one of the greatest health threats of the twenty-first century? In this chapter we'll see how CrossFit can help, not just in a general way, but in the life of an individual via a case study—Irene's story.

THE CROSSFIT SOLUTION

CrossFit coaches claim that CrossFit is *the* most effective program to combat obesity. They argue that this is because of the unique one-two punch of high-intensity exercise and nutritional principles in CrossFit. One: High-intensity exercise burns off weight and adds lean muscle mass more effectively than aerobic styles of exercise. And two: With its emphasis on a paleolithic-style diet combined with the Zone Diet, CrossFit attacks head-on the primary cause of the obesity epidemic in America: high-carbohydrate intake.

High sugar intake, as discussed in Chapter 5, is what rattles the insulin system of a human being into a state of hyperinsulinemia, a precursor to Type 2 diabetes. CrossFit coaches counsel members who have weight-loss goals to reduce their consumption of sugar, processed foods, and junk foods and replace them with the paleo-Zone foods: meat, chicken, fish, vegetables, fruits, and nuts and seeds in the right proportions. Starch and sugar are the enemy.

These theories make sense, but what about in practice? Does the program really work? In short, yes. And Irene's experience is a good illustration of how.

In my first few weeks at CrossFit Elysium, it quickly became evident to me that the ever-smiling Irene was the leader and central source of inspiration at the box. About 320 pounds at the time, she didn't exactly fit the stereotype of a CrossFit "star." But although the mainstream media often focuses its attention on elite athletes, CrossFit itself does not play favorites. It caters to the average person who is trying to get healthy and fit as much as it does to the award-winning athlete, and an average person, like Irene, can play as much of a role in the CrossFit community as one of the high-scoring members. If you visit a CrossFit affiliate during the day, don't expect to see a cadre of Special Forces soldiers working out; you're more likely to see a group of moms with babies and children in tow.

Irene is a powerful demonstration of the fact that CrossFit welcomes the beginner as well as the advanced athlete. Its ability to serve such a wide range of fitness levels is effectively tied up in two main dynamics. One of these dynamics is the two-way communication that takes place between coaches and athletes and between athletes and athletes. Every member of the gym has an active support system from day one. Coaches learn your name, you're introduced to the others in the gym, and you're treated as a member of the gym. The second is the structure that CrossFit uses whereby a competition-based workout is put into place each morning. This system allows people of all levels to, in effect, compete in the same race. Because of the competitive nature of the workouts, you are addressed as an athlete and referred to as an athlete.

These CrossFit dynamics turn the tables on a culture of watching and worshipping athletes on TV. CrossFit says that there is no reason we cannot define *ourselves* as athletes and live the athlete's life. It's a matter of showing up for it and making a commitment to it. Irene Mejia's story showcases this idea.

"I've been overweight my entire 38 years of life," Irene told me. "I'd pretty much tried everything. . . . NutriSystem, Jenny Craig, Weight Watchers, fad diets.

> **"I'VE BEEN OVERWEIGHT MY ENTIRE 38 YEARS OF LIFE," IRENE TOLD ME. "I'D PRETTY MUCH TRIED EVERYTHING."**

I may have lost a few pounds during each diet, but would quickly lose motivation and gain back whatever I lost plus some. About five years ago, I seriously considered gastric bypass surgery and started the process, but then my department was relocated out of state so I had no job, which meant no medical insurance. I was actually happy that I didn't have the surgery because deep down inside, I didn't want to do it that way, but at that time I felt desperate to lose the weight."

Irene had moved to San Diego from Los Angeles and worked for Kaiser Permanente as an account administrative rep for their accounts department. For six years, she also worked at Home Depot. During those six years, she worked, on average, 70 hours a week. Under that grueling schedule, diet and exercise became ever lower priorities, and her weight ballooned to 450 pounds.

The six-year slide could have had fatal consequences for Irene. Adult-onset diabetes was all but inevitable. She was also at risk for a slew of other health complications associated with morbid obesity.

"I finally ran out of excuses and started to take my health seriously back in January 2010," she said. "I cut out fast food and soda . . . exercised to a DVD, and walked on the treadmill about three to four times a week. I lost 45 pounds this way on my own from January 2010 to May 2010. I lost most of that weight in the first few months, but I started to notice my motivation slipping away the last couple of those months, and bad eating habits creeping back, and the weight began rising again."

Irene saw the sign for CrossFit Elysium during her commute and decided to check out the website. She e-mailed the coaches, one of whom was Leon Chang, to ask if it was possible for her to join.

A CAREFUL INTRODUCTION

Chang said that the first issue the coaches considered was Irene's range of motion—her ability to execute the movements. Her condition at the time was pretty extreme, and they needed to figure out whether CrossFit would be a suitable activity for her to try.

"When someone is morbidly obese, as Irene was, their ability to do CrossFit's full-body, compound movements is severely compromised," said Chang. He explained:

> Even body-weight movements such as an air squat may prove too challenging in the beginning. Indeed, Irene is still working on her basic mobility and range of motion to this day. She gets better with each workout, but still has a long way to go. We knew we were going to have to scale basically everything, whether it was range of motion, the weight used, or even the movement itself. As an example, when Irene started, she physically could not do a sit-up or a push-up. In both cases, she lacked the strength and mobility to execute the movement. In addition, both movements required getting her on the ground, and when she started, she physically could not get off the ground without assistance. So we scaled both movements (partial sit-ups lying on a bench, partial push-ups off of a bench), and as she's progressed, we've been able to get her doing both off the ground.

For the morbidly obese, Chang said, the range-of-motion problem is not simply a matter of deteriorated flexibility; it's a matter of sheer girth. "In Irene's case . . . her girth physically limits her ability to move in space," he explained. "For example, she can't touch her toes because of her belly, and she can't pull under the barbell well in a clean or snatch because it's too much girth to move through space. Similarly, she can't do a box jump because her legs, while strong relative to many of the other females in our gym, lack the ability to generate enough power to drive 300-plus pounds in the air to land on a box. So the daily challenge is coming up with movement substitutions or range-of-motion subs that will still provide the stimulus we're looking for, yet be possible for Irene to complete."

The coaches did not take the issue of welcoming Irene into their membership lightly; they talked at length about the dangers and obstacles her CrossFit regimen would entail. It was undoubtedly fortuitous that Irene chose a CrossFit gym that was co-owned by a medical doctor. Chang's insight into Irene's challenges derived from his medical background as well as from his knowledge of high-intensity exercise. In fact, in conversations with Chang, I was impressed with his knowledge and analysis of what CrossFit is and what it isn't. His study of the subject was very comprehensive, and because of his cautious, scientific nature, Chang was not your typical CrossFit "Kool-Aid" drinker. He worked and studied with coaches outside of CrossFit. As a result, when it came to implementation of policies, programs, and procedures at Elysium, his standards were high.

So the coaches strategized about how to meet the challenges of scaling the cardiovascular elements of CrossFit to Irene. Chang described their thinking in this way:

> We took it as a given that Irene wouldn't be able to handle intense exercise for long bouts of time. However, the self-scaling nature of what we do—push as hard as you can, go as fast as you can, but this is defined by you, the individual—meant that we just had to give her the parameters and guidance. Irene clearly displayed her willingness to work, so from the get-go, we knew we wouldn't have to worry about her slacking.

> The more worrisome possibility with the morbidly obese client is the existence of cardiovascular disease, joint dysfunction, or some other underlying health issue that will prevent meaningful exercise or even make exercise dangerous. There are no hard and fast rules here. All those "seek medical advice before engaging in any exercise program" bits that people see are worthless. No doctor can tell a person whether or not exercise is going to be 100 percent safe for him or her. In fact, the definition of what exercise even is remains open to interpretation: Is walking briskly three times a week exercise? What about carrying groceries? With so many unknowns, most MDs play it safe and

recommend the most sterile, least taxing form of activity for morbidly obese people. With this as an underlying attitude, something involving high-intensity exercise will certainly be regarded as "dangerous."

In some respects, it makes sense, because high-intensity exercise like CrossFit demands more cardiac output, creates more oxygen demand, and asks a lot more of a person's flexibility and joints than walking. Therefore, whether or not something like CrossFit is appropriate for the morbidly obese will remain an unanswerable question.

With Irene, I felt comfortable taking her on because, although she was morbidly obese, she was relatively young, being in her mid-thirties. She was "prediabetic" as a result of her weight, but otherwise had no risk factors for cardiovascular disease. So, we took her on and ramped her up slowly. If there were any signs her body couldn't handle what she was asking of it, we would have backed her off right away. Could I have demanded that she get a formal heart evaluation before taking her on? Sure, but in my analysis she was probably still low risk, and I didn't want to send her away—in which case the result would almost certainly have been she gets demotivated, never comes back, and ultimately does herself more of a disservice.

From her first months, Irene turned out to be an exceptional case. The same ethic that drove Irene to work 70 hours per week for six years was gradually rechanneled into CrossFit training. "The amazing thing is that Irene quickly proved her heart and lungs were up to the task," said Chang. "In fact, after a few weeks, she was regularly beating people in the gym, completing workouts faster or doing more rounds. If you think about the mass that Irene has to move and supply blood to, this is an even more phenomenal task. Not only is she often moving the same weight on the barbell as everyone else, but she has to move 100-plus more pounds of body weight as well. Clearly, her heart and lungs work just fine."

Chang was concerned about the level of motivation Irene would need to keep up for the long haul. It would take time to go from 450 pounds to an average, healthy weight. His wife, Dr. Alessandra Wall, a psychologist, specializes in working with patients with eating disorders. In those early discussions among the coaches about Irene, Wall brought up the realities of goal setting.

"I wanted to make sure they talked to Irene about her goals and encouraged her to be realistic in how long it would take," Wall said. "She would certainly go through plateaus, and it would be discouraging for her."

Chang agreed. "Motivation is a tricky issue with everyone," he said, "but especially morbidly obese clients." Time is the overriding factor: "The fear is that since they have such a long way to go, it's easy for them to lose motivation and quit when they're just getting started. A person who starts at 400 pounds and loses 100 is doing great, but they still may see themselves as a failure because they're still overweight. Similarly, if a morbidly obese person comes in not being able to do an air squat and after a year can do a passable overhead squat, that's a major accomplishment, but that person may not think they've achieved very much if they can only overhead squat the empty bar, and their neighbor can do 150 pounds."

Again, Irene proved an exception to the rule. The fact that Elysium was small worked to her advantage as well as she built a support network. Against the odds, she stayed motivated.

"Irene showed very early on that she possesses more motivation than perhaps anyone else in the gym," said Chang. "That motivation has been fueled by her continued fitness gains and weight loss, so it very quickly became a nonissue. In addition, the community at CrossFit Elysium is so supportive that she quickly made friends with many of the members, which is the most powerful motivating force one can have." Irene ended up not only staying motivated, but inspiring others. Photos and videos channeled through Facebook have taken Irene's story outside the boundaries of Elysium and to other parts of the country.

STARTING WITH FUNDAMENTALS

Let's try a thought experiment. Say you have heard the met-con horror stories, have seen the images on CrossFit.com, and have watched the videos and pictures of super-athletes executing all manner of seemingly impossible movements. You know about the pull-ups, the muscle-ups, the 50-inch vertical leaps onto towers of boxes and plates. And yet you have decided to bite anyway—you have made the decision to join a CrossFit gym and boot-camp your way back to health.

You know it's going to take some time. You know that as you walk in the gym, you'll be working out side by side with regulars who have V-shaped backs, parabolic curves to their quadriceps, defined shoulders, and vascular forearms.

Taking that first step into the gym might be a little tough. You might feel a bit of stage fright. But how much tougher would it be if you were morbidly obese? What if you were 405 pounds?

If you can imagine that feeling, you can begin to understand how Irene felt. "I was so nervous going to the first fundamentals class, I had butterflies all day at work just thinking about it," she told me. After the workout, she walked home. "It took me about three times as long. My legs felt like Jell-O so I had to take baby steps on the way back. There were even a few times my legs buckled underneath me. I had to grab hold of whatever was within hand reach so I wouldn't fall down."

> *"I COULD FEEL THE SORENESS WITH EVERY STEP I TOOK. GETTING UP AND DOWN FROM A SEATED POSITION FELT LIKE TORTURE."*

The next morning Irene's legs were deathly sore: "I could feel the soreness with every step I took. Getting up and down from a seated position felt like torture; I sat down on a low bench and it took me over 30 minutes to try to get back up. I was mad at myself for being so heavy—that I got so sore and couldn't even get up from the bench—and sad because I thought if this is how sore I'm going to be from doing the workouts, then there's no way I'm going to be able to physically do CrossFit."

A week transpired between her first and second classes, and by then the soreness had abated:

> I finished the fundamental classes in about one and a half weeks and was ready to start. Since my main focus was on losing weight and I knew this was going to be a long process, the first few months were the toughest. I started going about three times a week in the beginning, and I was extremely nervous each time. Though at the same time, I wanted to impress my coaches. I liked hearing their praise when I did a good job on a lift. Especially in the beginning, every week was setting a new PR because all my lifts started off just at the barbell. So I would get a high every time I PR'd. At the same time, I was starting to lose weight, so now I had proof that this was working. I remember in the beginning before every workout, I told Coach Paul, "Oh, I can't do that," and he would reply, "Yes you can." I became very familiar with the word "modify."

A very important factor for me in the beginning and to this day are the coaches themselves and my fellow athletes from Elysium. I love my coaches and my peeps from Elysium. The coaches worked with me every step of the way, and the other athletes made me feel so welcome.

REACHING FIRST GOALS

After 21 months of training at CrossFit Elysium, in March 2012 Irene reached a long-term goal. "I hit my under 300-pound goal on Sunday, March 18," she told me. "I was so excited. I usually would weigh myself Monday mornings and send a picture of the scale to the coaches, but I couldn't wait until that Monday. I had a good feeling I had already reached the goal, so I weighed myself Sunday instead. I was on Cloud 9 all day, actually all week long."

On the following Tuesday, CrossFit Elysium held a special workout in honor of her achievement. As a reward, Irene treated herself to a visit to Disneyland. "It had been about 15 years since I'd been there. I'd always been worried I wouldn't fit into any of the rides," she said.

Pictures showing how far Irene has come are nothing short of astounding. The sub-300-pound Irene is toned and radiant, with sparkling eyes and a huge smile. But it isn't just a matter of weight loss. In my conversations with members of Elysium during my time there, I found that the subject of Irene frequently came up, not only because she was a source of inspiration, but because she was someone they flat-out loved. Despite not being a typical athlete, Irene had become a leader at Elysium, if not a hero. Most likely, she would be considered both by anyone you might talk to there.

The coaches told me that Irene's success was as much a matter of her fierce determination as it was a result of the exercise and diet combination that CrossFit employs. But the exercise and diet combination was surely a powerful force. Rather than coming about as the result of a Weight Watchers-style calorie-counting program, working on the premise that weight loss is merely a matter of doing the math (expending more calories than you consume), the changes in Irene's body composition came about by a shift in body chemistry.

I asked Dr. Barry Sears to explain how the shift took place, and he explained what happens to the body in a case like hers when diet and training work in concert:

The weight loss is a consequence of hormonal changes that lead to the silencing of inflammatory genes as well as epigenetic changes. . . . In fact, a recent study has demonstrated [that] reducing carbohydrate while simultaneously increasing protein changes gene expression within 24 hours, with anti-inflammatory genes being up-regulated, and suppression of pro-inflammatory genes. The changes are maintained as long as the diet is maintained. If you put out the fire in the fat, then you lose the fat. Obviously a little more complex than calories in equals calories out.

In other words, when Irene started working out and changing her diet to agree with the CrossFit principles espoused by Sears, she immediately started the ball rolling for inflammation in her body to decline. Genes causing inflammation at the cellular level were suppressed. The expression of genes working against inflammation increased. And these changes all started within 24 hours. The result, as Irene persisted, was steady weight loss and muscle gain.

SETTING NEW GOALS

"My next goal is to lose another 50 pounds, to be under 250 pounds," Irene told me. "I also plan to lose these next 50 pounds much more quickly than the previous. I feel so energized and motivated, I am determined to reach that goal before the end of this year."

Irene's sub-300 achievement uncorked a new reservoir of motivation in her. She described to me her recent week of training: She had gone to six CrossFit WODs, and on five of those days she had added 2,000 meters of rowing to the WOD as "extra credit." She was also addressing two areas that had troubled her during the 21 months she'd been a member thus far: inconsistencies in her diet and insufficient sleep.

In terms of sleep, Irene had reported to the coaches that she averaged just five hours a night. They asked her to get at least seven. As for diet, Wall felt that Irene's progress had been slowed by issues in her attitude toward food that had not yet really undergone a big enough change. "The problem for Irene when it comes to diet is sustainability," Wall said. Wall believed that any long-term success in improving diet and health and in generating permanent weight loss had to be grounded in a person's fundamental approaches to food and cooking, rather than a no-holds-barred restrictive style of eating, or "detox"-like diets that count on elevated levels of willpower and day-in and day-out denial. "I'm not a huge fan of detox diets," Wall said. "I come from the notion that the more it fits into your everyday life, the more it will have a lasting effect."

Irene's basic routine had been to restrict herself to a diet of chicken and vegetables during the week, but on weekends to revert to old habits, which included lots of sugar and junk food. Wall realized that one of Irene's limitations in developing a more sustainable diet was that she didn't know how to cook. So Wall organized a series of get-togethers for some of the people at the gym. They would gather and spend an afternoon in the kitchen trying new, healthier recipes. The afternoons became a sort of workshop that allowed Irene to assimilate some basic cooking skills.

> MOST IMPRESSIVE WAS IRENE'S EMBRACE OF THE LIFESTYLE OF AN ATHLETE. SHE SIMPLY REFUSED TO ACCEPT ANY VIEW OF HERSELF THAT SOCIETY MIGHT THROW AT HER BECAUSE OF HER WEIGHT.

Irene's story continues. The new cooking skills may help her make progress even faster; to be the beneficiary of Wall's thoughtful cooking lessons certainly can't hurt. Nor can it hurt to have the kind of determination she has, or to have so many people warmly cheering her on. And she was lucky enough to find a CrossFit gym that not only had a doctor on staff, but a doctor whose wife specialized in eating disorders. All of these things have been working in her favor.

But how unusual is her story? Can CrossFit and CrossFit-style nutrition be an antidote for others who struggle with life-threatening weight problems? There is no one-size-fits-all answer to this question, as so much depends on the individual and the gym. The medical attention Chang was able to bring to her case was surely a necessary and crucial part of her success, and should not be left out by anyone in a similar situation who wants to try to follow in her footsteps.

Irene's courage was something to behold. Not only did she have the guts to come and join a CrossFit gym, but she has become the most active ambassador of CrossFit that I've met. She visits other CrossFit affiliates in the spirit of friendship and love for the community. She was also the catalyst at Elysium for throwing parties and putting together nights on the town for anyone who wanted to go. She corrals people into these events with a smile and a hug, and she will not accept no for an answer. Irene struck me as a one-woman campaign against antisocial isolationist behavior. I even got talked into going to a salsa dancing nightclub. This was not an easy thing to do.

Most impressive though, to me, was Irene's embrace of the lifestyle of an athlete. She simply refused to accept any view of herself that society might throw at her because of her weight. I worked out with her about twice a week, and at those workouts I often watched her battling to press large weights over her head or to push herself into the various states of being in "the pain cave" with met-cons. I watched her make breakthroughs: I saw her do her first burpee, and run 200 meters, when not long before that, she couldn't run five steps. And I'd watched all of this as the coaches treated her just the way they treated the others at Elysium. They expected 100 percent efforts, and nothing less.

An e-mail Irene sent to the Elysium coaching staff says it all. She wrote, "Even though I know I'm the heaviest one at the gym, I don't feel like the fat girl when I'm there, I feel like an athlete."

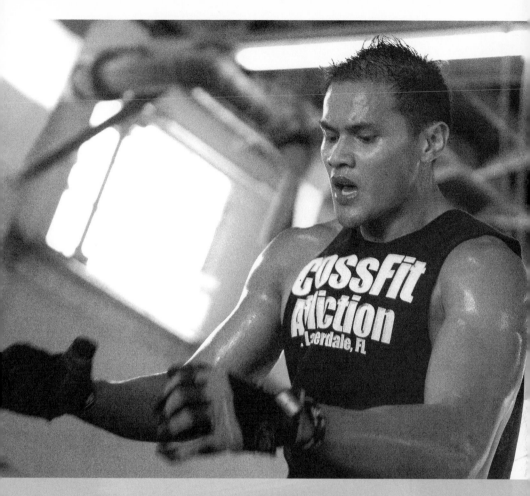

THE JET STREAM OF HIGH PERFORMANCE

THE MAKING OF A FIREBREATHER

"FIREBREATHER": 1. ONE WHO FACES THE TRIUMPHS AND TRIBULATIONS OF GREAT physical opposition with an indomitable spirit. 2. An optimistic energy associated with the heart of an athlete.

The use of this term in CrossFit dates back to the early years of Glassman's Santa Cruz CrossFit gym. It came about when Greg Amundson, a Santa Cruz sheriff with raw desire, discipline, and a full embrace of Glassman's instruction on topics ranging from training to nutrition, finished an especially brutal metcon, threw himself to the ground, and, in short, raspy breaths, said, "It feels like I'm breathing fire." Amundson was dubbed the first Firebreather, and the word was officially coined. Amundson, now a CrossFit coach, and others use it to designate CrossFit's fiercest members and the powerhouse CrossFitters who lead CrossFit affiliates.

But, as we've seen, metaphors abound in CrossFit, and the metaphor of fire alone is not sufficient to describe what brings CrossFit success; there is also a momentum that you can grab hold of, and for this we must turn to the metaphors of air and water. Glassman calls it the "jet stream of high performance." This powerful current propels CrossFitters to high levels of success. And, like any current, it waits there for anyone who decides to plunge into it. In CrossFit terms, that means anyone who has the discipline to accept the CrossFit proposition in total—and stick to it. The proposition in total is not just about training; it also includes sleep, hydration, paleo/Zone nutrition, mobility, and other ancillary disciplines. Ignore any one of them, and you are not getting the benefit of the full power of the CrossFit jet stream behind you.

Glassman's ideas about the jet stream seem true enough. From my observations, I would agree that anyone who commits to the total CrossFit lifestyle is able to make remarkable progress. But it seemed to me that it was also something else, this unique personality type, the firebreathing mind-set, that was common to all those who rise to CrossFit greatness. The Firebreathers are those who have figured out how to get into the very center of the current and harness its energy. They are able to achieve almost unimaginable feats of fitness.

The athletes I knew back in high school who most resembled firebreathing CrossFit athletes were the wrestlers—that is, in terms of discipline, not in degree of health. Indeed, wrestlers are known to live in a cyclic slash-and-burn world, where they repeatedly turn to weight-loss regimens to drop down to a weight class in the hours before a meet, and this is not a healthy habit. However, the attention wrestlers pay to the ancillary choices are similar; CrossFit becomes, for the cream of the firebreathing crop, a comprehensive lifestyle.

Words used to describe this personality type range from "driven" to "obsessed," and even "masochistic." It's difficult to describe the kind of person who is attracted to and excels at CrossFit—to come up with a psychological profile that is general enough to encompass the variety of people it should include while being specific enough to pin down what it is they have in common. What sticks with you most in watching Firebreathers is not simply the fact that they're good; it's the fact that they're driven. They've developed an enhanced capacity to suck it up and deal with high levels of discomfort on a consistent basis in order to go places in CrossFit that most people haven't even considered.

Every affiliate has its Firebreathers. Watching them, being around them at Elysium, motivated me to want to breathe fire, too. Their extraordinary efforts were on display in every workout, every day. However, it was in the competitions where they truly blazed their brightest.

THE THROWDOWN

In CrossFit there is an event that is known as a "throwdown," and it's climbing quickly on the radar of urban-adventure fitness aficionados. It's an informal back-alley "Fight Club" sort of competition, typically held at an affiliate gym with another local affiliate (or two) invited over for a day of competition WODs. There will likely be a team competition, open individual competitions, and a scaled category to open the door to all-comers. Roughly modeled on the CrossFit Games, the WODs are judged, and points are tallied as the competitors file through the day of WODs in heats.

The competitions have a festive atmosphere, with an almost barn-raising feel—people bring food and dogs and babies; they wear T-shirts and sweatshirts with their gyms' logos. Some members will be competing, and those who aren't will show up to cheer, scream, and mix with the fury of the music and crashing weights, creating a din that is worthy of the word "throwdown" and its nod to the "hoedowns" of yore.

The CrossFit Mission Gorge/858/Elysium Throwdown was held at CrossFit Elysium on November 12, 2011. It was a three-WOD event. Participating athletes would do each of the three workouts; their times would be recorded and they would also earn points. Unlike the CrossFit Games, where the athletes have no idea what the WODs are going to be until right before the start of the event, the workouts for the Elysium Throwdown were posted online in advance, with rules and standards for how they would be judged and scored. Although the competition was open to all skill levels (beginner-level participants could scale down workouts and have access to special judging), in order to compete for the open victory, competitors had to do the workouts as written and would be judged with a hard eye.

With a mixture of excitement and dread, I entered: excitement because I would be part of the team and enjoy the buzz of competing for points; dread because I'd seen enough of this stuff to know that by the end of the day someone might be carrying me home.

On the morning of the throwdown, I woke up nervous. I'd watched a throwdown several months earlier at CrossFit Mission Gorge. It was a heat-oppressed day in an overcrowded industrial space. Although the garage doors were open, it felt like you were in a jungle. The WOD I watched included three sets of 21 kettle-bell swings, 15 front squats, and 12 burpees, each burpee requiring a jump over the barbell.

I remember looking at the overwrought faces of the CrossFitters as their coaches and peers screamed at them to press on through the darkest moments of the 12-minute met-con. I could feel their pulse rates bob along above 200. They wanted to take just an extra breath of a break or a moment to chalk their hands. But this was exactly what their supporters were trying to thwart them from doing, intent on keeping the athletes from losing time or taking a dip in mental strength. If an athlete set down the barbell halfway through a set to rest, this set off a rally of imploring shouts from coaches, *"Get your hands on the bar. Get your hands on the bar now!"* For the athletes, there was no way to quit and nowhere to hide.

So I sipped my coffee and knew I was in for some of this sort of suffering. What had I gotten myself into? I'd felt this sense of foreboding before—when I'd entered an Ironman triathlon. I recalled the apprehension I had felt on that morning and noted that the apprehension was similar. You cling to the knowledge that because of the physics of time, it would in fact at some point be over.

READY, SET . . .

When I arrived, the gym was hopping. Almost everyone was clad in uniforms—sweatshirts, T-shirts, and beanies emblazoned with their gyms' names. Teams were clustered in groups on the front mat, athletes stretching and sprawled across foam rollers trying to loosen up. Several were working the rowing machines to warm up their muscles. Slow rap music played through the speakers, and the Elysium coaches were prepping the main workout area for the first WOD, moving 20-inch boxes into a line parallel to the row of pull-up bars.

On the south wall, heat sheets had been posted, and I went over to see what time I'd be going. There was also a printout of the WODs for me to study. This was the itinerary for the three workouts that day, with a long break between WODs #1 and #2 for about an hour and a lunch break between WODs #2 and #3.

The first WOD was a metabolic-conditioning "couplet"—a tag team of two exercises—and competitors would do As Many Rounds As Possible (AMRAP) within a given amount of time. A couplet can be any two exercises. In this case, it would be pull-ups and box jumps, and the allotted time for reps was 8 minutes. This WOD would test overall strength, agility, and stamina. In order to encourage all levels of CrossFitters to feel welcome in the competition, a scaled workout was also offered. This is how the instructions put it:

EVENT 1:
10 pull-ups, 10 box jumps (20 in.), AMRAP 8 min.
Scaled division: 10 ring rows, 10 box jumps or
step-ups (20 in.), AMRAP 8 min.

The second event would test the competitors' Olympic-weight lifting ability with the tried and true "clean and jerk." The clean and jerk is composed of two dynamic movements. In the first movement, you squat down to the bar and slowly lift it up until it's over your knees; you then "jump" the weight up by using power from the hips. Propelled aloft by the jump, the lifter then "pulls" himself underneath the bar and racks it under the chin and shoulders, from there extending upward with a front squat. Together, that's a "clean." You can stand there as long as you have time to stand there to catch your breath and prepare for the next move, which is "the jerk." The first phase of the jerk is a dip in the knees, which is like pulling back a short slingshot; then you channel the power of a hip snap to loft the barbell into the air a matter of inches. You get under the bar again, pushing up on it at the same time until you lock it out overhead, and then come to a complete standing position.

The clean and jerk is a rich, complicated skill that requires athletic ability, mobility, and speed as well as strength. This and the snatch (another Olympic lift, where you take the bar from the ground to overhead in one lightning-strike-like movement) are perhaps the most frustrating and difficult things to get a handle on in your first year. With WOD #2, competitors would have 8 minutes to work their way up to a one-rep lift from the ground to overhead with as much weight as they could possibly handle.

EVENT 2:

Max weight ground to overhead in 8 min.
Each athlete will have their own station with a barbell and weights to load.
Scaled division: same.

The third workout was the real reason I had trouble sleeping the night before the throwdown.

EVENT 3:

30 KB swings (M 53 / W 35 lb.), 20 burpees,
10 thrusters (M 115 / W 73 lb.), 3 rounds for time.
Scaled division: 30 KB swings (M 35 / W 26 lb.),
20 burpees, 10 thrusters (M 75 / W 53 lb.), 3 rounds for time.

Thrusters at 115 pounds, three rounds' worth, at the end of a day of WODs, not-so-delicately situated between burpees and kettle-bell swings. Each component of this workout involved compound movements that, when done in high numbers, give you the unmistakable feeling of having an egg beater spinning in your heart. For me, doing thrusters was one thing, but doing them with 115 pounds was another entirely. These were heavy thrusters.

A heat at a throwdown is actually a very orderly affair, despite the seeming chaos going on around it. Seven or so competitors would take to the floor, each assigned a judge. Judges were either members of one of the CrossFit gyms that weren't competing or other experienced CrossFitters or coaches from the San Diego community. The primary role of the judge is to maintain an official count of repetitions, counting only those that fulfill the "points of performance" as spelled out in the rules.

For example, if a competitor is doing a pull-up, but doesn't get his chin over the bar, the judge will say "No rep" and not count the pull-up. In a box jump, typically the jump will only be counted if the athlete fully extends the legs and hips when on top of the box. If you hop up on the box, landing with knees flexed, and never fully stand up, and then jump back to the ground, you'll hear "No rep," and all of that energy you just burned was for naught.

GAME ON

In the throwdown's first WOD, athletes lined up behind the pull-up bars. A crowd formed along the west side of the space and in a storage area above the space that was serving as a balcony. A rectangular digital clock hung at the east side of the gym, controlled by remote. Two waist-high containers of chalk powder were stationed in front of the black jump boxes.

Kipping pull-ups produce a lot of friction on the hands, and this being the first workout of three, with each workout requiring hands on the bars or kettle bells, athletes were wise to chalk up. The chalk reduces the wear and tear on the hands. A tear along the palm or at the base of a finger would ensure discomfort piled upon discomfort. By the start of the first heat, the air in CrossFit Elysium was already smoky with chalk dust.

"Three, two, one, go!" was the starting command for the first heat. Judging by the sinew of the competing CrossFitters, I estimated that two-thirds or so of the 36 competitors at the throwdown were the stronger CrossFitters from their respective gyms. At a typical class, I fell somewhere in the middle to top third of the group by that time. I quickly concluded that, today, my abilities were going to be in the lowest 25 percent of the group. With people howling encouragement from the back of the gym and from above, and the judges counting reps aloud, the competition began.

In my heat, I was between two fast athletes from other gyms, and I could tell through peripheral vision that my method for getting down off the box (I was stepping down rather than jumping down, which was legal under the rules) was costing me a lot of time. They were getting 1.5 to 2 reps for every one of mine. Plus, I had to break my pull-ups into batches of five at first in order to get a tiny break now and then. As the minutes rolled past, my fatigue built. By the middle of the heat, I could only do two pull-ups at a time; then I'd rest for a couple of seconds and go for another two reps. By the final two minutes, with my hands burning and my upper body emptied of energy, I was jumping up to grab the bar, rocking myself upward with a kipping movement, and barely getting my chin over the bar. That was all I had. I'd drop to the ground, let my muscles recover for a few seconds, and then repeat the process. My rivals at that point were also breaking up pull-ups, but they were still getting four or five at a time. The workout ended and I felt waves of fatigue and relief. I was one step closer to getting through this thing.

The second WOD was the clean and jerk, and here I betrayed my past as a runner. Long-distance running, as I had discovered in a humbling manner, tends to do a furniture-in-the-fireplace thing with athletic capacities like agility, mobility, and explosive power—all, as mentioned, critical to success with Olympic lifting. While the other guys were hoisting more than 200 pounds over their heads, I barely got 145, accomplished with a style one might see a sanitation worker use to hurl a bag of garbage into a truck. My judge explained the problem to me: I was trying to "muscle" the weight up; I didn't exhibit a trace of quality technique. And without technique (and with limited strength), you're just going to suck at Olympic lifting. This was an apt review of my performance at WOD #2.

It was time for the 90-minute lunch break. I ate my Tupperware lunch and braced myself for the discomfort to come in WOD #3. I was competing in the Open division, not the scaled division, which maybe I should not have done, because when I scrolled down the printout, listed in order of our current standings, to find my name, I had a hard time finding it, simply because it took me a while to scroll to the bottom. I was in last place.

The third and final WOD, #3, the death WOD. This is something you can expect at the end of all CrossFit competitions. The longest, hardest WODs are saved for last, when the athletes are already spent. At the CrossFit Games, the final WOD is called "Chipper"—named after a wood chipper—and it blasts the world's best CrossFitters with a broad collection of CF weapons that appear to be meant to slice the athlete up the way a chipper grinds a tree.

THE FINAL WOD

WOD #3 was composed of three classic compound movements: kettle-bell swings, burpees, and thrusters.

Here, some background information is in order: In addition to Olympic lifting, power lifting, and gymnastics, CrossFit has also assimilated movements from the rather obscure sport of kettle bell. Kettle bells were developed by Russian farmers as part of a weights and measures system for bartering grains. The iron bell was cast with a handle for easy transport. Community picnics among the farmers starting featuring strength competitions using the kettle bells, and a sport was born.

Iconic of CrossFit, the basic kettle-bell swing starts with the athlete holding the bell with both hands in front of her, arms hanging and fully extended. Then, using a thrust powered by the core muscles and hips, she drives the bell upward so that the KB swings to eye-level height or higher, depending on the standards the coach might have stated. If the athlete uses just her arms and shoulders for the KB swing, forget it—she won't last long. To do sets of 30 KB swings as dictated by WOD #3, you need to rely on core strength and power. And even then, 30 reps are going to tax you. In the case of this WOD, we were using 53-pound bells, known to Russian farmers as the 1.5 "pood" KB, which was defined by the Russian imperial weight system as equaling 24 kilograms.

Burpees, a.k.a. squat thrusts or up-and-downs, are another lung-burner, known well by American high-school athletes, particularly football players. If you're going to do CrossFit consistently, you'll do burpees at least once a week. They get planted into all sorts of met-cons to drive up the conditioning element in the workout. Twenty burpees in a round, following the KB swings, is a one-two punch in itself, teeing you up nicely for thrusters—the one-move combination of a front squat and a push press.

As I was in last place, I was in the first round, and was thus spared from having to watch the others get eaten alive by WOD #3. I would be part of the first wave of sacrifice.

My area was in the southeast corner of the gym, a small gift really, as the density of spectators was low there due to the lack of available space. Yet along the south wall, people were still two deep. I had my kettle bell, a space for burpees, and my 45-pound barbell loaded with two 35-pound charcoal bumper plates—115 pounds, which I knew from a quick look back through my training journal was more than I'd ever used in a single thruster. I knew that I should have tried to do a few to warm up, but I just didn't want to know what I already knew: Doing 10 reps of 115-pound thrusters was not something yet within my reach.

"Three, two, one, go." I broke the met-con up into pieces mentally, only thinking about what was immediately before me and suppressing thoughts on anything after that to try and rein in my level of emotional distress. This worked for the first two segments of the first round—through the 30 KB swings and the 20 burpees. I could hear my name along with words of encouragement from Elysium folk. Two segments down, I spun around and faced the barbell, squatted down, and performed a clean to get it to the front of my shoulders. I could see from the reaction in my judge's eyes—cold, unfiltered worry—that the clean was harder than it should have been. I then squatted down with the weight so that the crease of my hip was lower than the plane created by my knees and tried to explode upward. Begrudgingly, the weight moved. When it got to my chin, I drove it upward with a shoulder press and heard an odd sound come out of my mouth—like the sound a small mammal makes when it gets its leg clamped on by the teeth of a hunter's trap. My judge's eyes grew wide. The weights wobbled to the left, but I surged with adrenaline and locked out the lift.

HERE'S WHERE CROSSFIT GETS YOU: DESPITE THE COMMUNITY SPIRIT, ULTIMATELY IT'S ABOUT PERSONAL ACCOUNTABILITY AND DRIVING FOR GOALS THAT ARE MEANINGLESS TO EVERYONE BUT YOU.

With thrusters, you want to use momentum and rhythm to keep things chugging along. Ideally, the moment I had completed the rep, I would have quickly allowed gravity to suck the barbell back downward. I would have bent my knees with it as it sunk to the starting position. Instead, I had to drop the bar with a heavy bumper-plate crash to the ground. I could feel the eyes of the spectators around me—other CrossFitters who knew the state of my predicament.

I had 15 minutes to complete the workout, or, per the rules, I wouldn't officially finish. It was possible that the next 12 minutes would consist of me refusing to confront the fact that I had run out of power and continuing to try but failing over and over again to get through even just the first set of thrusters. My judge said, reassuringly, "Just take these one at a time." He knew the deal.

With each lift, I took three breaths, cleaned the weight to the shoulders, and went through the whole agonizing process again. As I worked my way through the first set, it felt as though I was reaching into my very intestines for some ghostly quality of energy. Each rep that I threaded my way through took a little bit more out of an emotional bank of energy. Somehow I managed to get through the first set. Sweat burned in my eyes. The muscles surrounding my chest couldn't keep up with the pace and expanse of my lungs. The crowd caught me breathing without working and told me to "pick up the kettle bell!" Round two began.

During the second set of thrusters, as I again took them one by one, a photographer shooting the event positioned himself between me and the garage door, which is the eastern wall of the gym. I don't think I can recall a moment in my life where I wanted to break the lens of a camera more than I did then.

The sounds I made during each rep became more and more embarrassing—high pitched and guttural simultaneously—but there was nothing I could do. I made it through the second set of thrusters and saw that I only had 4 minutes left of my 15 to officially finish the workout.

Here's where CrossFit gets you: Despite the community spirit, ultimately it's about personal accountability and driving for goals that are meaningless to everyone but you. It's not about awards or external recognition. It's about personal satisfaction. And because of the infinite variety of the workouts—the skills, drills, met-cons, WODs, Girls, Hero WODs, each with your own personal record attached to it—there's always *something* to agitate you into working to top your own record. This moment during the throwdown was one such moment for me—I might sure as hell finish last, but at that moment the only thing that mattered was the personal satisfaction of finishing the workout and recording an official time.

But by the third round, my body was cracking. I had to take the KB swings 10 at a time, and by the tenth rep of each 10, I was making agonized faces (caught by the camera, unfortunately) and creating new sorts of whimpering sounds. Burpees were my strongest suit and were just a matter of not stopping. But by the time I put my hands back on the barbell for the final set of thrusters, I had only a minute left. On my first attempt, I was able to thrust the bar above my shoulders about three inches, and then it just stopped moving and collapsed under the weight. I tried again and got one last official rep. The clock ran out and I was on the floor.

At that point I was just glad it was over.

ELYSIUM'S FIREBREATHERS

The final heat of the last WOD featured the guys who were leading in the scoring. I went to the balcony to watch. As expected, Elysium's Firebreathers shone brightly at the throwdown. One of them, Dave Bennett, was in the final heat and had a chance to win the men's event.

I watched him do the final WOD, the one I had struggled with. Elysium coaches Estrada and Chang hovered close to him, screaming almost constantly; they knew that if he won the workout, he'd win the overall competition. Dave spent the three rounds of burpees, KB swings, and thrusters in a space where he was simply outrunning most of the discomfort he was stacking up, putting all the pain on a physiological credit card by just continuing to move as fast as he could. Estrada and Chang kept up their barrage of words, a mixture of threats, orders, and encouragement. If Dave took even an instant of a break with the bar on the floor, the cries of "Dave, pick up the bar!" could be heard above the din of other coaches screaming the same things at their best athletes.

Having just lived through the workout as best I could, I found that it hurt to watch Bennett. He ignored the tremendous energy cost that he continued to demand from his body. When he finished the final thruster, winning the WOD and the overall, the bar smashed to the ground and he stuttered a couple of steps; in moments, he was lying flat on his back. All of the debt he had incurred tidal-waved him.

Bennett had been stationed in South Korea as well as Afghanistan with the U.S. Air Force, and he had discovered CrossFit while in South Korea. He had joined Elysium a few months after his discharge from the service. I had gotten to know him and had done an interview with him in the fall of 2011. So when I watched him lying on his back in victory, I was as proud as anyone there.

During our interview, he discussed what had attracted him to the sport. "CrossFit found me," Bennett told me. "I thought my fitness was unquestioned, then I met Tom Morrison. Tom was a 39-year-old TAC-P—special operations in the USAF. The first time I saw Tom, he was lifting weights from the ground to overhead with my one-rep-max 10 times, then sprinting 400 meters, only to repeat that couplet three more times." What he was seeing stopped Bennett cold. "Who was this guy? What was he on? Where do I get some?" he thought.

"That was the moment I left all other sports behind," Bennett said. He trained with Morrison for several months in South Korea, but then he was reassigned. His next duty assignment was in Colorado. He began training with Matt Hathcock, a personal trainer at a Bally's gym who was certified in CrossFit. Hathcock eventually started his own affiliate, CrossFit Unbroken, in Englewood, Colorado. "It was in this dingy, dim-lighted garage space that used to house a small taxi company," Bennett recalled. "We transformed that place into CrossFit paradise."

Dave is 5-foot-10, 175 pounds. His CrossFit numbers were solid: a 3:19 Fran, a max-pull-up total of 57, a 410-pound deadlift, and a 218-pound clean and jerk. He had not only become adept with the CrossFit movements, he had also built up a high level of pain tolerance, not unlike other Firebreathers. I became accustomed to seeing him come into the gym, straight from work, in dress shirt, tie, and slacks. The first thing he would do—methodically, and always before he even changed his clothes—was go to the whiteboard and examine the met-con. He'd also look to see how the other CrossFitters at Elysium who had come and gone throughout the day had performed; their scores, weights, and times were scrawled on the board by Coach Estrada.

In a CrossFit gym, rivalries surface between athletes of similar capacities. Vladimir Spasojevic was one of Bennett's friendly rivals—an exceptionally strong CrossFitter who usually worked out at 6 a.m. "Vladimir has no pain barrier," Estrada once commented. Bennett would see Vladimir's score and know that he'd probably have to push even harder than he had in the last workout in order to keep Spasojevic in line.

As Bennett lay sprawled on the ground at the throwdown, chest heaving for air, another Elysium CrossFitter, Karla Wagner, aware that Bennett was in danger of having a kettle bell land on his skull, talked him into dragging himself off to the sidelines.

Wagner, a Firebreather herself, would go on to win the overall women's competition at the throwdown that day. Like many CrossFitters, she was so fiercely devoted to the time spent in the box that it was easy to forget she had a life outside of it. In her day job, she was a public-health scholar and researcher at the University of California, San Diego. Part of her job consisted of making data-collection treks into Tijuana, where she interviewed prostitutes and drug addicts to establish correlates with the spread of HIV. I often wondered whether she brought her CrossFit toughness to bear at her job, or it was the toughness of her job that fueled her firebreathing at CrossFit. Either way, she was a force to contend with.

With short hair and sharp blue eyes, Wagner is lean but strong, with toned shoulders, arms, and legs, a physique shared by many of the more experienced and accomplished CrossFit women. They are about sinew rather than bulk—streamlined power. In the daily world of the gym, she had a stoic, quiet presence. I would see her offering encouragement to other gym members, but the words weren't given away cheaply. Rather, she always held them in reserve until the critical moments of a workout—a difficult lift for a PR, for example—and deliver them in almost a whisper. Says Estrada, "When she tells someone they can do it, or to not give up, it seems to be from a place of a coach, not a cheerleader." Other CrossFitters looked up to her. A word from Karla at the right moment could make all the difference between a disappointing "almost" and a chest-thumping

PR. Wagner, like Bennett, exemplified the style of internal leadership that the structure of CrossFit tends to make possible.

Bennett and Wagner are also both precision recordkeepers, noting their performances in workout logs on a daily basis. Their progress, or lack thereof, would be there in black and white. Bennett kept an Excel sheet where every CrossFit workout he had ever done had been recorded. Against this he set his goals. In our interview, I asked what goals he was working toward. He gave me two lists. One was for short-term goals, which were as follows:

1. Participate as a team competitor at the Games.
2. Get stronger: Squat 315#, Deadlift 415#, Clean & Jerk 235#, Overhead Squat 205#.
3. Work on flexibility (join yoga, Pilates, etc.).
4. Start an "outside the box" group from Elysium on Saturdays.
5. Become Level I certified and teach.
6. Stay healthy.
7. Do my best during Regionals for 2012.

Then there were the long-term goals:

1. Stay healthy.
2. Get others in a CrossFit box (friends, family).
3. Volunteer for CrossFit events.
4. CrossFit till death.

As I watched Bennett train over the course of a few months, I was able to see him directly attack these goals.

THE FIREBREATHING DIFFERENCE

Being a Firebreather is all about skill mastery. And in CrossFit, that means an ever-broadening array of skills, from core gymnastics movements, to Olympic lifts and power lifts, to various cardiovascular disciplines, such as rowing and running. The doctrine of CrossFit states that the program must be "constantly varying" in order to be effective. Herein lie both the reason for CrossFit's effectiveness and its biggest challenge. The CrossFitters who become Firebreathers unwaveringly pursue these skills, doing whatever it takes to master as many of them as they can—and especially those in which they are weakest.

The Crossfit.com main site frequently adds new, surprising elements to the training for the day. For example, one day the WOD included 25-meter underwater swims. (This was obviously not practical for all gyms, and franchises have the ability to modify the WOD, substituting another exercise.) At the 2011 Reebok CrossFit Games, competitors were tested in one event with how far they could throw a softball. Being prepared for the "unknown and the unknowable" is a major part of the overall programming.

Because there are so many skills to learn, the Firebreathers at a gym will typically add extra hours before or after workouts to work on skill development. They are the ones who show up early for a workout and stay afterward. I had observed this in Bennett and Wagner. Other members at the gym might do some light stretching or massage their backs with a foam roller before a workout. Bennett and Wagner would be far more aggressive, using a "glute-ham" developer machine (which looks like a medieval torture device) to perform back extensions, or gymnastics rings to do ring dips or work on their muscle-ups.

In his warm-ups, Bennett performs tactical assaults on all of his "goats"— a term for the weaknesses that have been revealed to a CrossFitter in workouts. Kelly Starrett also calls them "holes in performance." Identifying goats, Starrett says, is one of the primary reasons an athlete should train in CrossFit. "If the gym is the lab, we're in a controlled and safe environment. This is where we can spot the holes in performance that are holding you back."

One of the few times I saw Bennett struggle with a goat was when part of the workout included "pistols." A pistol is a gymnastics move, a demanding and complicated form of a single-leg squat requiring exceptional balance, strength, and flexibility. Bennett agonized over the move during the workout, but then he made it the focus of his warm-ups. That kind of head-on confrontation with one's weaknesses is something that sets Firebreathers apart from other CrossFitters. A non-Firebreather in his situation might want to avoid the headache of doing pistols again. Maybe they wouldn't come up in another workout for a while, the non-Firebreather might rationalize. Maybe he could skip a WOD where they did come up. Given the constantly varying WODS, it's fairly easy to let a skill or two remain your goat. Bennett, however, made working on pistols part of his daily ritual.

When I asked him about this, he shrugged and said, "That's what I do whenever I come across something I suck at. I make it part of my warm-up." Whenever I come across this level of determination and single-mindedness of purpose in someone, it always makes me feel just a little bit lazier. Nevertheless, I had great admiration for that kind of attitude, and for Dave Bennett for having it.

After workouts, both Wagner and Bennett continue their skill work. Many times they can be seen back on the gymnastics rings, working on muscle-ups. Muscle-ups are a defining move in the CrossFit world, but they are also a classic goat. There are those who have them and those who don't, and they seem to be the unofficial divide between beginners and the advanced.

HEAD-ON CONFRONTATION WITH ONE'S WEAKNESSES IS SOMETHING THAT SETS FIREBREATHERS APART FROM OTHER CROSSFITTERS.

Both Wagner and Bennett not only worked consistently but hard. On weekends, they often competed in events like the throwdown. They also were regulars at the Sunday morning CrossFit Elysium "Elite" WOD—a 90-minute session requiring advanced skills and fitness. They would go hard day after day, but then, when they'd had it, they'd take complete rest days. This ability to back off seemed to me to separate them from compulsive exercisers I have known, who have a hard time listening to their body's cues and resting. It also reflected yet again an exceptional sense of discipline and control.

"I listen to my body," Bennett told me after a particularly brutal met-con. "Right now I'm just whacked. Just destroyed. So I'll take tomorrow off. I'll take off two or three days if I need it."

Wagner, too, built in time for recovery. At Elysium, on Wednesday nights, I joined her in a yoga class that followed the workout. I noticed one night that she was trying to turn off the competitive, achievement-oriented side of herself. During one particularly difficult position, made more difficult by the fact that this was following a particularly difficult WOD, in which there had been both a max-strength move and a met-con, the teacher noticed Wagner's frustration and asked if she was okay. "I'm just trying to not get all aggro over this," Wagner replied. She wanted—really needed, she said—the yoga to be an hour of her day when she could turn off the goal-pursuit side of her brain and relax.

Despite this careful attention to recovery, with the number of hours each was logging at the box, some wear and tear was inevitable. A Firebreather's hands—in particular, the palms—are where this is most evident. Both Bennett and Wagner took great care of their hands; both spent time meticulously taping their hands before workouts—with ringlets of tape around vulnerable fingers. "Tearing"is what it's called when friction incurred during pull-ups leaves a spliced finger or palm— or an entire callus comes off. In one of my late-night CrossFit.com binges, I came across a video of a guy with the look and demeanor of a Viking who wore a crazed grin as he tore off a long strip of skin from his hand. Shredded and bleeding hands are not uncommon, and calluses are worn with a kind of pride. In my first months as a CrossFitter, with my hands slowly adapting to the new stress, I once lost a callus and found myself in a fandango of trying to heal the tissue, contain infection, and stop the pain. I wasn't thrilled over it, but in a way it felt like part of the initiation.

Pull-ups did the most damage, but damage to hands is also a problem when it comes to kettle-bell swings, Olympic lifts, toes-to-bar exercises, and work on the rings. In something like the CrossFit Games, where athletes are doing two or three long workouts a day for three days, the hands require even more care than usual. At CrossFit Elysium, it was not uncommon to see Coach Estrada, a Firebreather in his own right, and the shape and size of an NFL outside linebacker, standing casually in a corner of the box, filing down the calluses on his hands. Bennett uses sandpaper. All use hand lotion.

LEARNING HUMILITY

Dave Bennett's willingness to face his goats day after day; Irene Mejia's decision to take her first step into a CrossFit gym; my own humiliating experience the first day I attended a CrossFit class and could barely perform an overhead squat, where it was clear to all just how far I had to go—in a way, all these things were teaching me the same lesson: To get to the upper crust of the CrossFit landscape, you have to have humility.

When navigating your way through the layers of intensity and the myriad skill levels, there's just no way you can progress without learning that lesson. You're not going to avoid—sometimes, and probably many times, especially at first—getting left behind in a workout. At the CrossFit Elysium Throwdown, I looked at the results the next day and was hit with the news that among those who didn't scale the workouts, I was dead last.

I grew up playing football and basketball and running track, and eventually I became a good marathoner and decent triathlete. I'm pretty certain that the throwdown was the first time I'd come in last in anything I'd willingly entered. That takes some getting used to, and I'd be lying if I said I didn't care that the numbers were so public. But it is that very element, at least in part, that helps fuel personal growth in CrossFit, turning an average athlete into a Firebreather. I shrugged off my last-place finish because, for one thing, I knew it wasn't going to be the last time it happened. But it was also because, as I looked at my score, and those listed atop mine, I could feel the flame inside of myself burn just a little higher. I was already thinking about the next throwdown.

TO GET TO THE UPPER CRUST OF THE CROSSFIT LANDSCAPE, YOU HAVE TO HAVE HUMILITY.

In an article about CrossFit for *Men's Health* published in October 2011, writer Grant Stoddard wrote about how he tried CrossFit, but didn't take to it. He thought maybe he just wasn't that attracted to a fitness movement where people posted videos of themselves exercising. And Stoddard is right—many CrossFitters love to post pictures and videos of themselves on Facebook and YouTube. That said, I know distance runners who would happily post videos of their running races. As a matter of fact, some elite runners from yesteryear, such as Kenyan Henry Rono, formerly a holder of multiple world records, seem to do a lot of this on Facebook.

Anyway, I don't think that's what got to Stoddard. I think he didn't like the sport because, as he reported in his story, the women in the class simply torched him in a workout. I know the feeling. I had it the first time I went in, I had it when I came in last at the throwdown, I had it when I trailed behind an athlete who was making it even harder on himself by wearing a weight vest, for crying out loud, and I imagine that just about everyone who has ever worked up the courage to go to a CrossFit class for the first time has had the same experience. Everyone gets creamed, and not only gets creamed, but has the facts of their getting creamed put on display next to their name on a whiteboard.

How a person responds to that experience says a lot. It suggests how he or she might ultimately do at CrossFit. Some people who attempt it will vanish quickly, as Stoddard did; others will hang in there for a while and learn not to worry too much about where they rank, finding their spot in a CrossFit community where they just don't let it get to them.

And then there are the ones who will gravitate toward that jet stream of high performance. These are the ones who are motivated because they didn't like getting beat, but who have the tenacity to keep going back. They may be getting beat every day, but they are also getting a little bit better every day, systematically attacking their weaknesses, until, one day, they discover they've become a Firebreather.

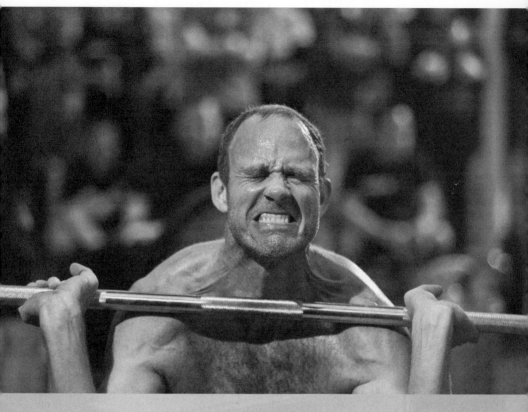

MY DATE
WITH FRAN

9

NOVEMBER 18, 2011. ELEVEN A.M. CLASS AT CROSSFIT ELYSIUM. FRIDAY. COACH
Paul Estrada in the house. I was there at 10 minutes to the hour. The met-con of the day was "Danny"—a 20-minute AMRAP Hero WOD of 30 box jumps, 20 push presses, and 30 pull-ups. The workout was named after Oakland SWAT Sergeant Daniel Sakai, 35 years old, who had been killed on March 21, 2009, in the line of duty along with fellow officers Sergeant Ervin Romans, Sergeant Mark Dunakin, and Officer John Hege by a convicted felon wanted on a parole violation.

I warmed up on the Concept2 ergometer rowing machine, an easy 500 meters to loosen up the shoulders, the trunk, and the back. It made a pleasant whirring sound. Five minutes 'til, and I was still the only one who had shown up for the class. It reminded me of something Greg Glassman had discovered in the early days of CrossFit when he had shifted his personal training business from one-on-one coaching to a small-group model. He would charge each client less, but he would ultimately make more money in the hour. He also watched with curiosity and amazement as it became clear that his clients preferred the groups to going solo. Why? he wondered. Likely it was because, in a group, the attention is spread out, and with the high-intensity, high-discomfort form of training Glassman used, not having his full attention every minute of the workout seemed, to his clients, like a benefit. It took off some of the pressure.

Estrada, too, is a great coach. He is skilled at saying just enough to keep you giving a total effort. There are hyper-enthusiastic CrossFitters and CrossFit coaches, but Estrada is not one of them. In terms of praise, "Less is more" is his policy. Or maybe "Least is best." He is ruthless, in a caring way, and has tremendous vision; in classes, he has the uncanny ability to see into and gauge the effort of every athlete.

Estrada, 6-foot-4 and towering from above, generally stood in a corner with his arms crossed, for the greatest field of vision possible. His head did not move, but his eyes scanned the room, back and forth, harvesting details to criticize or positives to reinforce. The larger the group, the more serious his tone. What I would most often hear was, "Get your weight on your heels"; "Keep the bar close to your body"; "Knees out"; "Elbows up"; or "Keep moving."

Estrada's voice was usually firm but calm. If he saw anything hinting at laziness, his voice would rise. Particularly vicious met-cons, which would essentially knock the legs out from the entire class, generated no warm-and-fuzzy reactions from Estrada. Whining about how hard the workout was netted exactly zero reaction. A classic scene at the end of a CrossFit Elysium workout was a room of supine bodies gasping for oxygen, legs and arms askew, Estrada just standing in the corner, arms crossed like a security gate, his brown eyes offering not a wisp of sympathy.

So the point? Having the attention of Paul Estrada spread across a group seemed to strike the right homeostasis. Being the only one in the class could be rough on the ego. I began to brace myself for the experience of having Estrada's pace of critical observations having nowhere to go except toward me.

As the clock turned from 10:59 to 11:00, Estrada turned to me and then looked at the whiteboard, considering the workout that was scheduled, and considering that it would be no big deal to change it, since I was the only one in the class. I knew what was coming. I could feel cortisol releasing into my bloodstream. Muscles clenched around my stomach. My senses shifted into battle-ready status. I could hear a delivery truck outside whine into second gear. I pulled down on the sides of the knit stocking cap that I had bought at Disneyland, burgundy, with a Mickey Mouse patch stitched to the front. All of the traditional fight-or-flight stress systems had simultaneously leaped into action, increasing my heart rate, blood pressure, and rate of breathing.

"How about Fran? Want to test it today?" Estrada asked.

"Sure, yeah. That's a great idea."

TEST-RETEST

"Test-Retest" is a big phrase in the CrossFit world. Have doubts that a diet works, or the overall training philosophy or programming? Want to see double-blind, peer-reviewed research to support the ideas, but it just doesn't exist? The CrossFit answer is to try it yourself and see if it works for you or not. Test, retest.

1. Test: Get a reading on your current fitness level.
2. Try the program for a given number of weeks.
3. Retest.

That November, I wanted to test the antispecific training doctrine of synthesis, the idea that the best way to train for a specific CrossFit goal is with general CrossFit training. Just wake up every morning, go to the gym, do the

WOD that's on the board, eat good food, get lots of sleep, drink enough water, then retest to see how far you've come.

Four months into my life as a CrossFitter, I'd heard several tales of success using this process—how someone had a deadlift PR, and even though he rarely did a deadlift in the course of two or so months, he retested a one-rep maximum deadlift and posted a serious gain.

This flies in the face of the conventional training rules I'd grown up with, in particular the principle of specificity. That principle states that the way to move toward your athletic goals is to do your thing. If your goal is to run faster, then run a lot. If it's to bench-press more weight, do a lot of bench presses. If it's to jump high in the air, jump a lot. What CrossFit tries to teach you is that the best way to attack a CrossFit goal is to just do the general training.

If there was one aspect about CrossFit that I believed was bullshit, this was it.

To be fair, this principle is intertwined with the notion that the ultimate goal of CrossFit is a broad state of general fitness and health. Coaches I spoke with on this subject acknowledged that, yes, if you just want to improve your Fran time, then just doing thrusters and pull-ups in every workout is going to be a fast way to do it. But you'll become a sort of "fringe" athlete in the process, someone who is especially good at Fran, but ultimately regressing in everything else. The extreme example in another sport is the high-mileage marathon runner who trains solely for marathons, essentially leaving certain other types of athleticism (agility, for example) to the margins. Everything is sacrificed in the quest to run a long way at a swift pace.

The CrossFit model encourages the athlete to set goals and then pursue those goals with an intensified focus on doing all the basics. For example, say you've been going to CrossFit three times a week, but you've paid little attention to the things you consider "extras," like nutrition, mobility, and sleep. You work with a coach to set a goal, or a set of goals, and look to reach them by being a better CrossFitter. A beginner might set goals like these:

1. Lose 5 pounds of fat.
2. Master an unassisted pull-up.
3. Lower 500-meter rowing time by 10 seconds.

Maybe you're expecting a nutrition plan, to go with goal #1. And various exercises that would target #2, along with a lot of rowing. But that is almost assuredly not what you would get. Instead, the coach might set up a plan for you that would across the board require a higher level of commitment. It might be an eight-week plan that requires you to make it to CrossFit four times per week. The coach might also set various benchmarks for improving nutrition (as you expected) and getting more sleep (something you may not have expected). You might have to do some extras in your warm-ups that touch upon specific goals (such as practicing your pull-up), but you would not be given specific workouts. There are no specific workouts. There's just the daily drumbeat of the ever-varying WOD.

A side note on sleep: I asked Coach Chang, who is an MD, to explain to me why sleep is so important to CrossFit training. "Most of us are sleep deprived," he said. "This translates into an inability to recover fully from both life's routine stressors and physical training. With lack of sleep, the gains one would otherwise make from working out are blunted, and progress is slowed." Chang also said that lack of sleep increases cortisol levels, a stress hormone that decreases immune function. It also, he said, "inhibits thyroid function, which slows metabolism and decreases caloric burning, causes fat deposition in the back and abdomen, and also . . . breaks down muscle and connective tissue."

Okay, he convinced me about the sleep issue. But I still had my doubts about the efficacy of nonspecific training. So I decided to do a test-retest. I wanted to see for myself whether this theory worked.

SETTING THE GOALS

Coaches Estrada and Chang came up with two key goals for me, chosen from among the classics in the CrossFit world: improving my Fran time and upping my max deadlift. The goals were spread across broad time and modal domains; in other words, I was going to focus on two different types of exercise that ranged from taking very little time (upping my max deadlift) to taking relatively more time (bettering my Fran).

Fran, probably the best-known CrossFit workout, and famed for the puke-seducing amount of internal discomfort it delivers, tests not only strength and power but also stamina, coordination, mobility, and mental strength. The deadlift, on the other hand, is more of a brute strength sort of thing. Say a tree trunk falls and traps your friend, and you have to use all your strength to get it off him. The deadlift is the most effective way, using just the human body, to save your friend. A max one-rep deadlift attempt has never made me want to puke, but it does involve a huge amount of blood being plunged by the working muscles; and the slish-slosh of systolic and diastolic blood pressure that occurs when I try to stand up after that always tags me with a galactic head rush. I wobble around the gym for about 20 seconds, dazed by vertigo.

Performing a deadlift takes at most a couple of seconds, but in those few seconds, it makes a huge demand on overall physical power. Fran, in contrast, is done by the best CrossFitters in three minutes, possibly faster, but might take a beginner half an hour. Beginners usually don't have the strength or the skill to do the kipping pull-ups and thrusters that Fran comprises. These components require strength, power, and exceptional mobility in the hips and shoulders. Both kipping pull-ups and thrusters make excessive demands on large muscle groups, such as those surrounding the hips and shoulders, generating a tremendous amount of power. The power usage comes at a cost, however, as after you've ripped through a high number of kipping pull-ups or thrusters, your respiratory system feels like it's veered to the edge of implosion.[1]

Fran's notoriety lies in the sharp blow of metabolic discomfort that it delivers to the athlete. That's why the phrase "For a good time, call Fran: 21-15-9" is the quintessential CrossFit T-shirt, the secret handshake, and the official rite of passage.

"So why don't you get your bar set up," said Coach Estrada. "And get a medicine ball, too." The medicine ball was to be set so that each thruster I performed went to the proper depth; in order for a rep to count, every time I got to the bottom of the movement my butt was required to make contact with the ball. The

---

1. I was once talking to a track coach who was also an exercise physiologist, and he relayed to me a story about a legendary exercise physiologist and track coach that relates to the intensity involved in workouts like Fran. The story may have been apocryphal, but it is worth telling. Apparently the legendary coach was in the lab with a coaching intern and called him over to a large bucket of water. He wanted to show the young coach how much effort and training effect he could demand out of his runners in a track workout. The old scientist-coach then dropped a rat into the water, and the rat had no way out of the bucket. It just had to swim or try to swim to stay alive. The two watched the rat struggle for a while, and then, as it began to tire, it began to drown. When the rat was giving into the exhaustion, the coach grabbed it by the tail and saved it, holding the thoroughly drained rat up for display purposes and saying, "That's exhaustion." One of the things that happens in the first weeks and months and maybe years of doing CrossFit is that a CrossFitter who continues to push goes beyond what he or she thought was possible in terms of exhaustion and discomfort. If you don't continue to push forward, then progress will inevitably come to a stale halt.

other point of performance was that the bar would have to be fully extended and my elbows locked out at the top. The pull-ups required that the chin get over the bar on each rep and that the arms lock out at the bottom of the pull-up.

The plan was to do Fran as a pretest; after 10 more weeks of CrossFit, I would retest. The same would go for a maximum deadlift. I had already tested my deadlift earlier that week, and my one-rep max was 295 pounds.

Estrada pulled up a chair and set the digital clock at the rear of the gym to stopwatch mode. It would be 21 thrusters, 21 pull-ups, 15 thrusters, 15 pull-ups, 9 thrusters, 9 pull-ups.

By the time of the pretest, I could do kipping pull-ups, so I would be doing that part of the workout as prescribed. The fastest CrossFitters prefer the butterfly pull-up, where the body pattern is reminiscent of how a swimmer does the butterfly. My choice would be the more common kipping-style pull-up, where the body uses core muscles in a horizontal push-pull motion to create energy to go upward. Once you get the pattern going, there's a powerful momentum to be gained and used toward higher numbers of pull-ups.

> **FRAN'S NOTORIETY LIES IN THE SHARP BLOW OF METABOLIC DISCOMFORT THAT IT DELIVERS TO THE ATHLETE.**

But my capacity with front squats and push presses—the two elements of a thruster—was still lacking, so Estrada suggested I do the workout with 75 pounds—still 20 shy of the prescribed weight.

"Three, two, one, go," Estrada said. To get an elite time, an athlete needs to do the thrusters and pull-ups as close to "unbroken" as possible, meaning that you don't break up the sets. For example, you don't break up the first 21 reps into one set of 10 and one set of 11 with a short rest where you quickly catch your breath. I, however, would break the sets up a lot, especially as the workout wore on. Although I was able to break the first set of pull-ups into only two batches, by the third set I was doing them one by one.

Estrada encouraged me to try and get two at a time, but when I couldn't get them, he just tried to keep me moving by limiting the breaks to durations as short as possible. "Get back on the bar," he said over and over. When you're standing there late in the workout, on the verge of ventilatory overload, your chest feeling like a gas can into which someone has dropped a lighted match, getting your hands back on the bar becomes a harder and harder thing to do. But at the same time, you realize that it's going to hurt no matter what, so you might as well get it over with as fast as possible.

I finished the Fran pretest in 8:20 and experienced for the first time the great Fran backlash–that when it's over, it's not really over. The point at which you feel your absolute worst after Fran occurs maybe a minute or two after it's done. I had my hands on my knees and was staring at the ground, and then I had to sit down on the floor, it got so bad.

"Jesus," I said.

"No," Estrada replied. "*Fran.*"

10 WEEKS OF TRAINING

The 10 weeks of training for the retest commenced the next day. It was a simple plan: Go to CrossFit classes four or five times per week for 10 weeks, with stretching/mobility exercises before and after classes. Drink a lot of water, eat good food, and get eight hours of sleep per night.

Attending class four to five times a week fell in line with the CrossFit philosophy on attendance. The ideal pattern, it holds, is either three days on, one day off, or five days on, two days off. Dave Castro, codirector of training, says this is the basic line of thought, but that an athlete should always remember that "routine is the enemy," and so, whatever you do, mix it up. Constantly vary the pattern. So in addition to the 3:1 or 5:2 schedule, throw in a three-day recovery once in a while, or four consecutive days of training. Keep your body guessing.

At the top of the CrossFit world, you'll find athletes keeping schedules that reflect a high level of dedication—and pain tolerance. Lindsey Smith, for example, of Columbus, Ohio, one of the top women CrossFitters in the world, often does two workouts a day. What is especially impressive about this is that she's not napping between workouts, to say the least. Smith is a wife, a mother, and a schoolteacher, and she travels most weekends to teach at CrossFit certifications. I asked her about that second workout of the day. She admitted that sometimes she didn't get a chance to do it until late at night after her daughter was put to bed.

"Well," she said, somewhat matter-of-factly, and with a light shrug, "You just do it."

In my case, getting to CrossFit four times a week was all I could handle. Sometimes I went five times a week during that 10-week training period; however, I noticed that I was a physical wreck at the end of those weeks. I was also not much fun to train with. Once, on the fifth consecutive workout in a week, I showed up and the met-con included power cleans with heavy weight, one of my weaknesses. We were teamed up in groups of three, and while one person did the set of power cleans, the other two rested. My teammates saw that I was struggling and tried to cheer me on. I responded to their kindness by swearing and slamming the weights to the ground. Not great for team morale.

I decided that, in general, after four consecutive days, I was so spent that it was counterproductive to go in on the fifth day.

JUDGMENT DAY

Monday, January 30, would be the Fran retest.

As the day crept closer, I grew more nervous about it. For one thing, I was afraid I was going to prove myself right about CrossFit and do worse than I had the first time. It just didn't feel like I was training for what I was going to be tested on. Only once during that period had I encountered a workout with thrusters in it. So how was I going to get better at thrusters, the key component of Fran? I didn't feel like I was making any radical gains in my ability to do pull-ups, either. It seemed like the 10 weeks would go by and I'd retest Fran and be lucky to be able to complete it. The same went for the deadlift: I spent very little time doing the exercise. The fear that I would fail at both goals became vivid.

I was also nervous because I knew how much Fran was going to hurt. I knew my desire to improve my time would be great, and thus I knew Fran was going to get real ugly, real quick.

I asked original Firebreather Greg Amundson, who has more than 10 years of CrossFit workouts under his belt, how many times he'd done Fran. "More than 100," he replied. He told me that in the early years of CrossFit, when he traveled with Glassman to teach groups what CrossFit was all about and do certifications, he was often so nervous the night before an event that he couldn't sleep. He knew he would be called upon to blow himself to pieces by doing Fran.

The early certifications had loose schedules, so he wasn't even sure when the Fran demonstration would take place. "I would never know when it was going to be," he said. "It could be in the morning, it could be after lunch. It could be during lunch. I had no idea." In one CrossFit.com video, Glassman talks about how knowing you're going to do Fran is almost as bad as doing it. He says he has seen elite CrossFitters so anxious about Fran that they threw up *before* the workout.

The stress that Amundson felt before such workouts ultimately pushed him to adopt a sort of in-the-moment philosophy, where he would divide the world into the things he could control and the things he couldn't control. Amundson realized that he could only truly have an impact on the present moment, and that worrying about what may or may not happen in the future—when he would be told to do Fran—was beyond his control. Letting anxiety sap his energy was a waste. He has since become the official "goals" coach for CrossFit, teaching specialty seminars at CrossFit affiliates around the country with this philosophy as one of his main topics.

I tried to apply Amundson's technique as the end of January approached. The Fran retest was only a week away. Estrada broke a bit of protocol by telling me that he'd help me a little bit by programming Fran into the schedule. "Don't miss the Monday workout," he said.

On the whiteboard that day:

STRENGTH
Thruster 3 x 3

MET-CON
"Fran" for time
21-15-9
Thrusters (95/65)
Pull-ups

While a sub-4-minute Fran is highly respectable, a sub-3-minute Fran puts you in rare company. As of this writing, the men's 2011 Reebok CrossFit Games champion, Rich Froning Jr., has a personal record of 2:17 for Fran. Kristan Clever, the women's 2011 champion, has recorded a 2:49 Fran. Chris Spealler, from Park City, Utah, who has an otherworldly personal record for max pull-ups (106), has a 2:07 Fran PR.

And then there's Jason "Rhabdo" Kaplan's 1:53 Fran, recorded at CrossFit Montclair in Montclair, New Jersey, and posted on YouTube in May 2009—perhaps the most watched Fran in the history of CrossFit. From the corner of a cinderblock gym, Kaplan walks into the picture wearing a long-sleeved black shirt, long gray shorts, and wire-rimmed glasses. Within the frame of the video is the digital clock that is timing him. From the beginning, Kaplan's efficiency is thorough. Not only is he breathtakingly quick with the 95 pounds of weights—it pops so lightly into the air you'd think the bar was unloaded—it's obvious that he's refined the entire workout to trim any waste. On the completion of a set of thrusters, after the bar literally pops into the air before dropping, a testament to the speed and power being employed by Kaplan, he doesn't even turn around but instead takes two steps backward to get to the pull-up bar. The bar looks like it's set perfectly for his height. As his legs swing through the butterfly pull-ups, they look like they're an inch off the ground. It takes Kaplan just 48 seconds to get through the 21 thrusters and 21 pull-ups. By 1:28 he's completed the 15-rep round. At the finish of the 1:53 Fran, CrossFitters from the gym spill into the image and congratulate the freshly flattened Kaplan, who cries out, "No more Fran! Never again! No more!"

STICKING TO THE PLAN

I called up Amundson to ask for his advice on my Fran retest. He offered me two ideas to improve my performance. Amundson told me to be sure to organize myself at the outset with the equipment; time is precious, so don't waste it shuttling back and forth between the pull-up bar and the barbell. He said to look for every possible way you can tweak the situation to save time. He also advised planning breaks in advance. For example, I could plan to break the 21 thrusters up into 11 reps and then 10 reps, putting the weights down, and taking a specific number of breaths while transitioning to the pull-ups. "Even if you feel especially good, don't throw away the plan and try and get the set all in one," he said. "Stick to your plan."

Although thrusters and pull-ups had received no special attention in the 10-week period of training, I had made two important discoveries along the way. One was a breakthrough with the kipping pull-up. One day during a met-con, all the mechanics of it snapped into place, and the idea that momentum would propel me over the bar, like a swing, finally took hold. Whereas before I had struggled to use the kip to get over the bar, now it felt closer to the way it looked when I watched the others do kipping pull-ups.

In addition, the one time we did thrusters in those 10 weeks, Estrada had given me some sage advice. He had taught me how to do them faster, again by capitalizing on momentum. Once you lock out at the end of a thruster with the bar overhead, he said, you quickly squat down so the weight can just sink with gravity, rather than trying to control it and burning energy. I also had a better feel for using the power generated by snapping the hips to propel the bar upward. The most common bad habit for beginners is to try and muscle the bar up with each thruster using the arm muscles. Using these smaller muscles, which aren't nearly as powerful as the muscles of the hips and core, and will flame out much faster, is a sure way to perish before the workout is over.

FINISHING THE 15 PULL-UPS GIVES YOU THAT "LIGHT AT THE END OF THE TUNNEL" FEELING.

Fran. It was 11:44 a.m. We'd spent the class so far working up to a maximum amount of weight for three thrusters, and now we'd set up our stations for Fran. Coach Estrada was joining in on the workout. Usually Estrada is stoic, whether coaching or training, but this time he was pressing his forehead into one of the building's support beams with a sort of delirious smile on his face. "This is going to hurt," he said softly, and tried to laugh.

The clock started and we were off. I was again using 75 pounds, as in my first test, which meant I was still doing a scaled workout. However, Chang had told me that the lighter weight didn't mean that I would be getting away with anything. "You'll be able to go faster, so it may even hurt more than if you were using 95 pounds."

I used my new technique of letting the weight come down fast and folding down underneath it. The first 21 thrusters flew by. I broke the pull-ups into two sets: 11 reps, down for three breaths, then 10 reps. I returned to the thrusters for the 15 reps. Breathing and heart rate were high. The discomfort is a weird sensation. It's centered in the chest and abdomen, as if the internal organs are getting the worst of it. It's kind of a searing feeling of sickness.

Finishing the 15 pull-ups gives you that "light at the end of the tunnel" feeling. Now you just go as fast as you can without the muscles failing you. The great ones—Amundson, Smith, Kaplan, Spealler, Sakamoto, and others who can go under 3 minutes—don't break anything up. I, however, had to do the last six pull-ups one at a time. I'd leap onto the bar, kip a pull-up, let go, come back down to the ground, and immediately jump back up.

I'd also broken up the last two sets of thrusters. But with Amundson's and Estrada's advice in mind, I kept my breaks as tight and controlled as possible. Estrada finished well before me—his Fran PR is 3:01—and was now coaching me and the others on, mostly keeping us focused on containing breaks to a bare minimum. I finished and slumped to the floor. A wave of metabolic fatigue washed through me and I felt sick. But the discomfort was eased by the time I'd clocked.

On November 18, 2011, in the pretest, my time had been 8:20. My goal had been cautious: I wanted to break 8 minutes. My time on January 30 was 5:27. I'd cut nearly 3 minutes off my Fran time. I was astounded. It had been 10 weeks. A year before this, I had been a limping mess of damaged gristle. There was no denying that, for me, CrossFit's antispecificity training worked.

I also retested my max deadlift that week. Two and a half months before, I had PR'd with 295 pounds. In the last week of January, we did the one-max-deadlift test. Wearing weight lifting shoes and gripping the cool steel of the 45-pound bar loaded with a total of 315 pounds, I had a new PR.

This is how they get you, I realized. It is this march toward personal records, goals, and programs, checking new skills off the list, making new records, seeing gains in strength and endurance, losing pounds of weight or fat. Being able to do a pull-up or being able to "RX" a workout. This is the drug that gets you—and keeps you.

EPILOGUE

THE FUTURE OF CROSSFIT

IN EARLY MAY 2012, I WAS IN CEDAR RAPIDS, IOWA, TO VISIT FAMILY. I WENT TO work out at CrossFit Cedar Rapids, a small box located near a movie theater complex on the northeast side of town. Justin Lowinski was coaching. I asked him how business was.

"It's great," he said. "When I started coaching here, just about one year ago, our largest classes had maybe 5 or 6 people in them. Now we're getting over 20 people per class." Lowinski said they planned to open up another affiliate in June to handle the demand.

In April I had talked to TJ Belger, co-owner of four CrossFit gyms spread out in Marin, California. Although Belger's original personal-training gym—before he discovered CrossFit—was on the verge of going out of business, since affiliation he has expanded it to the four boxes, and they're thriving. The only "problem" they've struggled with is how to meet the growing demand. "We have 1,000 members now," he told me. "And the classes are starting to max out."

In terms of sheer numbers, CrossFit Elysium in San Diego is another example of CrossFit's rapid march upward. When I started in July 2011, Elysium had 50 members. The gym had just moved, because its membership had outgrown its space. During the next six months, I watched as membership doubled. People would join the gym and start getting fit, and their friends would ask, "What are you doing?" The friends would then come to try a workout at Elysium. It was too much for some, and they'd disappear. For others, it was love at first workout, and they became an integral part of the community.

At an affiliates' gathering in Big Sky, MT, in a talk caught on a CrossFit.com videotape, Glassman acknowledged that some gyms have become incredible financial successes. "We have million-dollar-a-year boxes out there," he said. "Boxes that bring in more than $100k per month."

CrossFit is continuing to grow despite a critical fact: CrossFit is not for everyone. I've seen plenty of people try it and leave it behind. Some don't like the group dynamic; others don't want to trade in the meditative aspects of steady-state jogging or biking, or yoga. Others don't want to be inside a gym at all and want to pursue outdoor activities. That's all more than understandable. But what's happening is that CrossFit is reaching the people who love it.

And with growth, change is bound to take place. Some changes are already on the horizon. What will corporate involvement mean for CrossFit, for example? How will demographics affect it? How will the loose-knit style of the affiliate system play itself out? Is CrossFit in danger of being "tamed" as it ages? Is it in danger of being diluted by sheer growth?

On a sunny Saturday morning after a rain-drenched week, April 28, 2012, standing on the gritty blacktop at San Francisco CrossFit, if I turned and faced north I would be looking at the Golden Gate Bridge, the Marin Headlands, and Crissy Field. If I turned around I'd be looking at a fleet of cranes and construction crews that were demolishing Doyle Drive, an elevated road that connected the Golden Gate Bridge to central San Francisco. The roar of the jackhammers and the grind of the diesel engines drowned out the rap music the gym was playing through outdoor Insignia speakers. I was doing burpees next to a SFCF storage container on the pale pavement of the parking lot. It was hot and I was sweating, my hands chafing from the burpees. It had been a foggy, rainy spring, and the sun had drawn a lot of members out for the morning.

> **BUT WHAT'S HAPPENING IS THAT CROSSFIT IS REACHING THE PEOPLE WHO LOVE IT. AND WITH GROWTH, CHANGE IS BOUND TO TAKE PLACE. SOME CHANGES ARE ALREADY ON THE HORIZON.**

Before I started my workout, I was watching the crews beat apart the highway. The coach, Angel Orozco, a SF native who was wearing a hooded SFCF sweatshirt and sunglasses, saw me in my moment of awe and joined me to watch.

"This," Angel said with a broad smile, looking at the crew of athletes working out with the backdrop of the demolition, "is what CrossFit is all about."

I understood what he meant. Unlike most of the world, which seemed hellbent on selling you immediate gratification, pleasure, and comfort, here was a place that offered only one deal: You get out of this what you put into this. There are no secrets. Jim Baker, one of Greg Glassman's first CrossFitters, says that Glassman didn't invent anything new—rather, he organized effective exercises within an effective strategy. The centerpiece was hard work, pain, and sacrifice propelled by a group dynamic.

This was the template set in Glassman's original Santa Cruz gym. They didn't need peer-reviewed studies published in sports medicine journals to know it worked. They knew it worked because the athletes in the gym got faster, stronger, and more powerful—and these were areas of athleticism they could monitor with a stopwatch. They transformed their bodies into superhero-like physiques.

The ethical code that is the DNA of CrossFit was built on this respect for a persistence-pays-off, no-bullshit, no-frills approach; it was a statement of anti-luxury and anti-convenience and anti-softness. For people who were sick of slick marketing and false promises and decadence, the innovation and existence of CrossFit offered a connection to others who felt the same way.

Part of the attraction of CrossFit has been that it has an underground mystique to it. It has been, thus far, a community bound together through a grassroots irreverence for the megacorporations that seem to have an unshakable grip on American society. So an underlying fear within the CrossFit community, of course, is that growth and popularity will lead to its ruin. What if CrossFit got sold to one of these megacorporations just interested in maximizing revenue?

In 2010-2011, fear of this scenario was fueled when a multimillion-dollar, 10-year sponsor partnership between CrossFit HQ and Reebok International was signed and the sponsorship began to affect CrossFit.com programming. The CrossFit Games became the Reebok CrossFit Games. A gym culture that had had a back-to-basics theme in terms of equipment, shoes, and clothing was now the target of a company selling CrossFit T-shirts for $48 and baseball caps for $28. Videos showcasing Reebok products and Reebok people started getting featured on CrossFit.com.

A great shudder was felt through the affiliate community. Had CrossFit sold its soul to Reebok? Was it going to become encapsulated by the shoe giant known for its historical connections to "Step" classes and aerobics? Was CrossFit.com going to try to shove pro-Reebok videos—marketing thinly disguised as news pieces—down the throats of CrossFitters? An angry throng reacted on the forum boards. Was this the beginning of the end?

I spoke to one longtime affiliate owner in Orange County and asked him what he thought of the Reebok contract. "I'll tell you this: The day they tell me

I have to call my gym a Reebok CrossFit gym is the day I drop the word CrossFit from my gym's name."

According to Reebok representatives and CrossFit HQ, that's not in the plan. However, Reebok is opening up its own affiliates, which are branded "Reebok CrossFit." Reebok representatives say that most of these boxes will be outside of the United States, in accordance with a plan to break into different countries. They also suggested there may soon be opportunities for existing gyms to receive loans to upgrade in exchange for adding "Reebok" to their name.

Reebok corporate leaders spent a year getting to know the CrossFit culture and introducing it to their employees. In July 2011, I paid a visit to Reebok's headquarters outside of Boston and "CrossFit One," a box and training facility for Reebok employees. I went to a noontime class, and it was packed—there were maybe 30 employees doing the WOD. The facility was state of the art. This was no garage gym, for sure. And there were three coaches pacing through the ranks throughout the workout.

I met some powerful spokespeople for CrossFit at Reebok, including one employee, Peggy Baker, who is 53 years old. Baker has type 2 diabetes and has been working for Reebok for 27 years. She only tried CrossFit because she wanted to be able to tell her employees that she hated it. But the support she received from a Reebok CrossFit coach and the other participants in that first workout was so overwhelming that she got choked up just recounting the story to me. She continued with CrossFit, and since then, she has lost 33 pounds. Her diabetes has begun to recede. When I asked her what she had to say to others who were struggling with diabetes and weight problems, she replied, "If I can do it, you can do it."

One thing is for sure: The exposure of CrossFit through ESPN broadcasting of the Reebok CrossFit Games will pour gasoline on the fire of CrossFit's growth. This will only add to an already furiously expanding business, one that has been built almost entirely on word of mouth. Reebok commercials featuring CrossFit workouts and athletes have also begun to add to the mainstream exposure.

Greg Glassman doesn't appear to have any interest in letting CrossFit be taken over by Reebok or anyone else. CrossFit HQ is staffed by many people whom he has known for years and who came out of the original gym.

Glassman no longer coaches at a CrossFit box, and he no longer teaches seminars or even shows up at them ("I become a distraction," he says). When asked about what a typical day is like for him, he says he spends a lot of time on the phone, talking to lawyers and insurance people, but he doesn't try to micromanage the evolution of CrossFit. It appears as though Glassman's current obsession is with penetrating new areas with CrossFit that will yield positive results in situations where results can be quantified.

"I don't have a lot of far-reaching visions for five years," Glassman said in a *CrossFit Journal* video in 2011. "Much of it is just reactive." Perhaps unsurprisingly, Glassman explained that he looks at it from a numbers perspective, seeking patterns. "It's a view from 60,000 feet and you look and say, what the fuck is that? It's changing rapidly. We encourage the good ideas and discourage the bad ones."

One passion that Glassman has that the CrossFit world can expect to take shape in coming years is a data-collection project being driven through Vor Data Systems, a science and engineering company that specializes in extracting data from complex systems and multiple sources. The idea is to collect data from sources like the CrossFit Open and the Reebok CrossFit Games and to be able to give quality scientific predictions about the consequences of different actions. How did the dinner you ate today affect your health? How does doing a particular kind of workout influence your longevity? This hard-wrought data will contribute an enormous amount of valuable information to the discussion about diet and exercise. In talks Glassman has given on the subject, it's apparent that the Vor Data Systems project is critical to the development of his 3D model of health, where an athlete can chart power output (fitness) over the years. With the brand of data collection Glassman has in mind, he believes that questions that tend to inspire emotionally charged answers—questions like, "What's the best diet, paleo or Zone?" or "What's the most effective exercise? Aerobic or anaerobic?"—can be answered by crunching the numbers.

> GLASSMAN'S CURRENT OBSESSION IS WITH PENETRATING NEW AREAS WITH CROSSFIT THAT WILL YIELD POSITIVE RESULTS IN SITUATIONS WHERE RESULTS CAN BE QUANTIFIED.

In the next 5 to 10 years, another aspect of CrossFit that will likely change is its clientele. For example, while my first impression through CrossFit.com was that the movement catered to men, the doors have clearly been thrown open to women. More than once I've been one of the only males in a group dominated by large numbers of women.

Glassman has talked about how, over the years of his coaching, one of the more profound patterns he believes occurs is that women gain confidence through CrossFit training. This, he says, directly translates to advances in their careers. One woman at Elysium, in her early twenties, told me that before CrossFit she would have never been found doing any sport, except for yoga. "I never felt comfortable in gyms because of all the guys staring at you," she told me after a workout. "But there's something about the community here that makes it comfortable to work out with guys. I actually like it. The weirdness is gone."

In addition, much of the CrossFit clientele is now 20- and 30-somethings, but aging Baby Boomers are already beginning to discover it in droves, and even CrossFit kids' programs are sprouting up throughout the affiliate system—I've now seen classes of 3- to 6-year-olds up through the teenage level. One of Glassman's new passions in terms of extending the CrossFit community into schools is combining fitness training with an SAT preparation course for teenagers. And despite any impression one might get from the CrossFit Games, which might indicate that CrossFit is for Olympian-like youth, CrossFit, with its functional aspects, is well suited for seniors. Being able to move, get up and down steps, retain overall mobility and health—these are goals that CrossFit can help people with as they age. Jim Baker of Santa Cruz CrossFit specializes in working with athletes who are age 60 and above. When he begins working with a new client in that age group, he makes sure his on-ramp program is performed at a welcoming intensity. Even if a new 70-year-old client can do a full squat, Baker will start him out with a quarter-squat and work to slowly build momentum and confidence.

As Baby Boomers, officially those who were born between 1946 and 1964, come to CrossFit, there will be no shortage of clients. Baker believes this is a good thing. "Ten thousand people turn 65 every day," he said. "What I want to say to affiliate owners is: You have these gyms that are largely empty during the middle hours of the day. You can be training retired people then. They're incredibly loyal members of the gym."

Baker adds that seniors are incredibly disciplined, as well. "They don't miss workouts because of hangovers." Plus, there's the fact that the doctrine of CrossFit is to encourage people of all levels of ability, so even in the classes with younger athletes, a senior CrossFitter should feel welcome.

"There was a point at Greg's original gym when he was transitioning from coaching individuals one-on-one to the classes," Baker says. "Well, I was doing the

WOD and I was 30 years older than others who were doing the workout. They finished the WOD and could have gone out and had a coffee and come back before I was finished. But there they were, clapping for me and helping me finish."

That's the true spirit of it all. The future of the movement depends upon it.

For my part, I have undergone changes (and revelations) of my own. My interest is now in uniting my experience with CrossFit into my love for running. Before I joined CrossFit Elysium, I did a six-week program that introduced me to Brian MacKenzie's CrossFit Endurance program. The heart of the program is transitioning to the Pose Running Method.

Two to three times a week, I did drills and short sprints that were meant to rewire my foot strike, my body position, and the muscles I was using to run. For me, this meant changing from heel-strikes and hip-flexor power to midfoot running and power from the hamstrings and glutes. It also meant paying attention to my cadence, following MacKenzie's technique of using a metronome to set my pace. Week by week, my cadence became quicker. At first, it was incredibly tiring, even for short drills. But by week three, it started to click. I began to feel like my legs were moving like wheels. By the end, I was running 200- and 400-meter intervals at paces under six minutes, a speed I hadn't been able to touch for years because of being hobbled.

So I was making progress. But with so many weaknesses and holes in my strength, I decided to focus just on CrossFit for a while. This is about to change. In the next year, I'm planning to really work on integrating CrossFit into a running program. I'm curious to see what this effort will yield. For me, it's a whole new world.

GLOSSARY OF TERMS

AMRAP: Acronym for "as many rounds as possible" completed in the time allotted for a workout. Pronounced "am-wrap."

Box: A CrossFit gym.

CrossFit Games: A competition among the world's best CrossFit athletes and teams, spread out across several days. Most of the contests are announced only within a week of the Games; some are not revealed until the very day of the contest.

CrossFit Open: The first qualifying phase of the annual CrossFit Games. It is open to all and judged at an affiliate or through submission of a video. More than 60,000 people entered the 2012 Open.

Firebreathers: The top athletes at a CrossFit affiliate. Firebreathers are the performance leaders at the box.

For time: Term applied to workouts that must be completed as quickly as possible, with few, if any, breaks in effort.

Girls: Foundational CrossFit workouts that, like hurricanes, are named after women.

Globo gym: What CrossFitters call typical big-box fitness centers.

GPP: Acronym for General Physical Preparedness, which is a primary aim of CrossFit training—to prepare the user for a wide variety of athletic challenges, as opposed to specific events.

Hero workouts: Particularly long and tough workouts named after fallen soldiers, firefighters, and police officers.

Met-con: Shorthand term for a metabolic-conditioning workout, the iconic high-intensity element of CrossFit training that trains stamina and endurance.

MOD: Shorthand term for modifying a workout to make it attainable. (*See also* **scaling.**)

Nasty girls: A popular online video of three early stars of CrossFit—Annie Sakamoto, Eva Twardokens, and Nicole Carroll—performing a benchmark workout of air squats, muscle-ups, and power cleans at the first CrossFit gym in Santa Cruz. It is widely noted as inspiring many to join CrossFit.

PR: Personal record. Most benchmark WODs are set up to produce maximum levels of effort by encouraging athletes to beat their personal bests to show overall improvement. PRs are also kept for individual lifts, like the deadlift or the clean and jerk.

Pukie the Clown: CrossFit's mascot. A "visit from Pukie the Clown" means that you've vomited following a WOD.

RX: The prescribed requirements for a WOD.

Scaling: Lowering the prescribed weight or changing the exercises to make a workout accessible to beginning or intermediate CrossFitters.

Sweat angel: The imprint of sweat left on the floor after a WOD has blasted a CrossFitter.

WOD: Acronym for "workout of the day." Pronounced "wad."

GLOSSARY OF EXERCISES

AIR SQUAT

From standing position, descend to bring your hips below the knees » Press knees outward and track them over the feet throughout » Keep torso upright and arms extended » Return to standing position

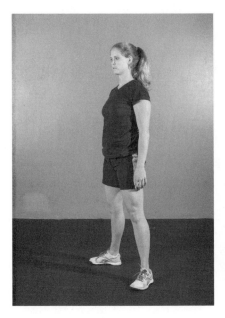 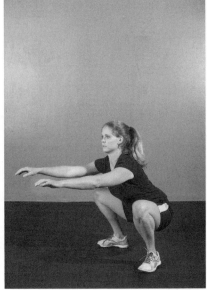

BALL SLAM

Stand with ball overhead **»** Throw ball to floor using power from core **»** Catch ball in squatted position

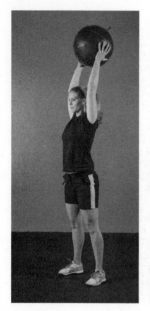 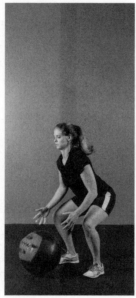 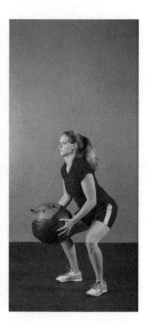

BOX JUMP

Stand facing box » Jump onto box » Fully extend body and lock out knees » Jump or step down

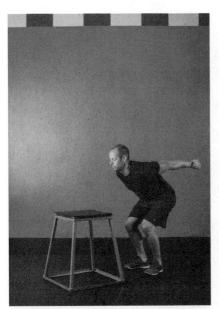 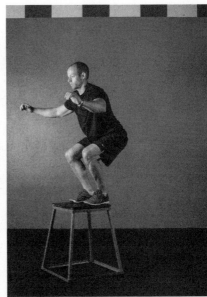

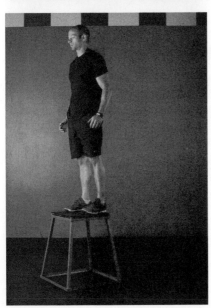

BURPEE

Start from standing position » Squat down to floor » Spring legs backward and drop into push-up position » Touch chest to floor » Complete push-up » Return to standing position » Jump up and clap hands over head

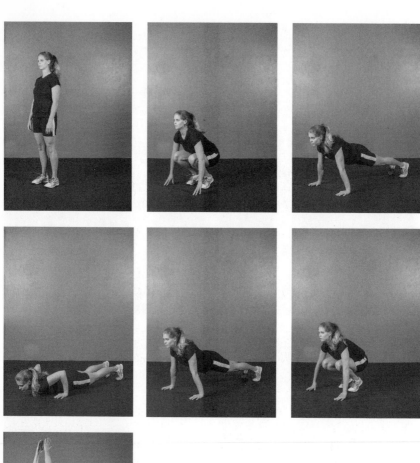

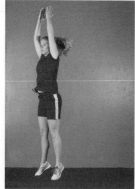

CLEAN & JERK

Grip bar on ground, knees shoulder-width apart, back straight, knees bent ❯❯ Lift to rack position on front of shoulders ❯❯ Dip and thrust weight upward ❯❯ Split legs to drop down underneath the bar ❯❯ Lock out arms with weight above and stand

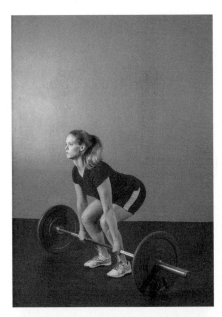 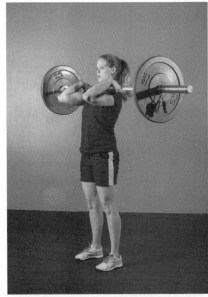

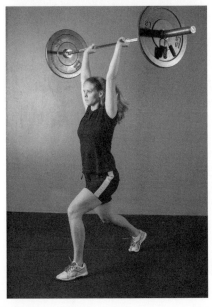 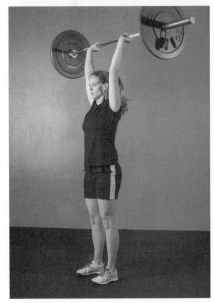

DEADLIFT

With good lumbar position, grip bar from the ground » Lift weights to hip-level with full extension

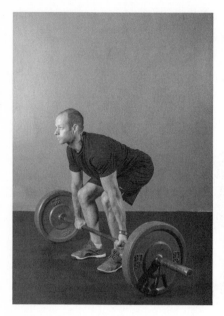 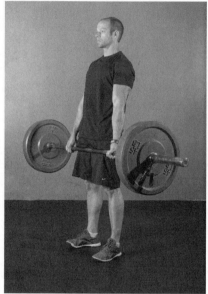

FRONT SQUAT

Rack bar beneath chin on front of shoulders » Squat with hips dropping below knee level » Press knees outward and track them over feet throughout » Return to standing position

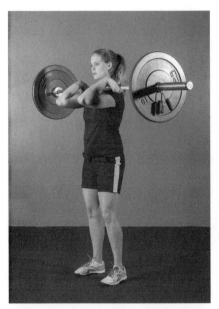 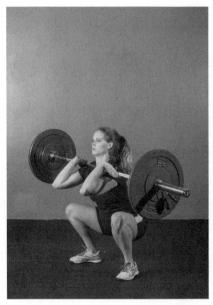

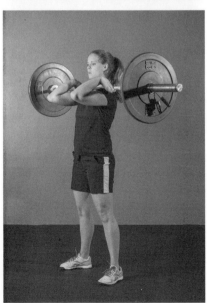

HANDSTAND AGAINST WALL

Assume handstand position with feet against wall **»** With core tight, bend arms at the elbows and drop head to floor **»** Return to handstand position

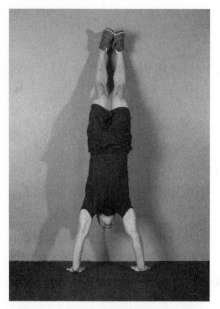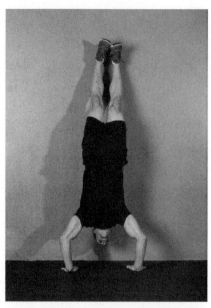

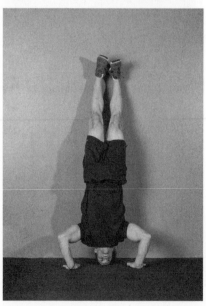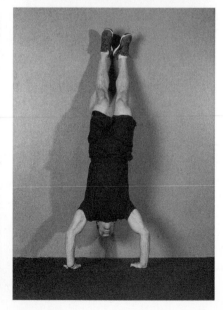

KETTLE-BELL SWING

With knees bent, grip kettle bell with both hands and tighten core » Use hip drive to swing the kettle bell upward » Return to starting position

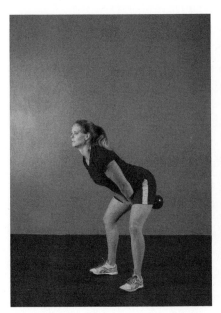
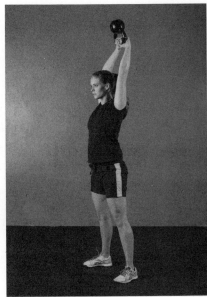

KIPPING PULL-UP

From hanging position on pull-up bar, activate shoulders to generate horizontal swing » Use hip and shoulder power to move body upward with chin clearing the bar » Keep core tight as you press away from the bar and channel momentum back into the swing

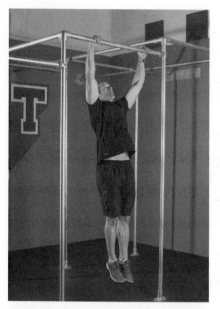 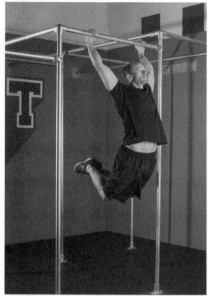

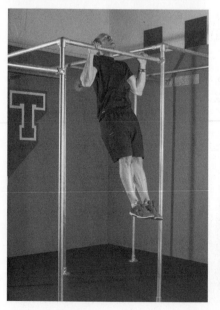 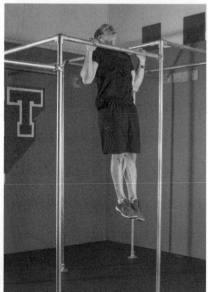

MEDICINE-BALL CLEAN

With weight on heels and upright torso, knees bent, grip the ball on the ground » Using hip drive, thrust ball to shoulder-rack position » Drop down to squat position » Return to standing position with ball in shoulder-rack position

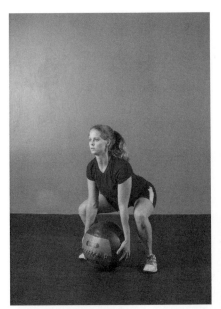 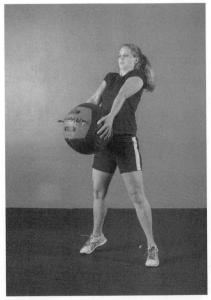

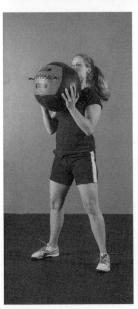 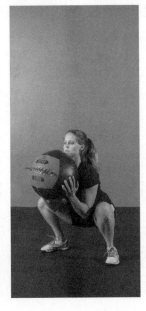 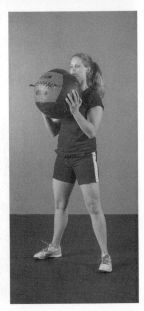

MUSCLE-UP

Hang from rings **»** Pull up into press position, with elbows bent and legs straight out in front of you **»** Press up to full extension

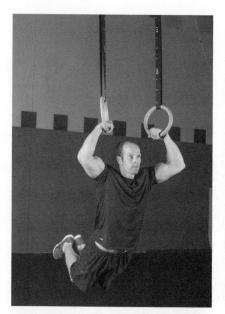
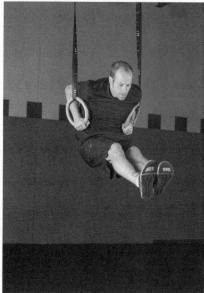

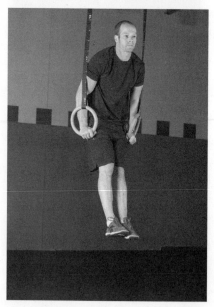

OVERHEAD SQUAT

With wide grip and bar extended overhead, perform full squat **»** Keep core tight and track knees over feet throughout

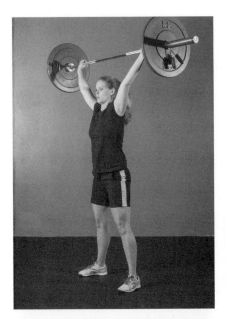

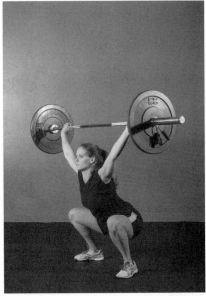

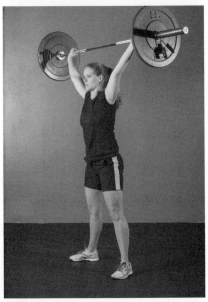

PRESS

Stand with feet shoulder-width apart, weight racked on front of shoulder **»** Keeping knees locked, press weight above head **»** Return to starting position

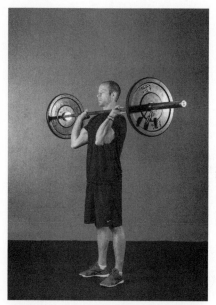 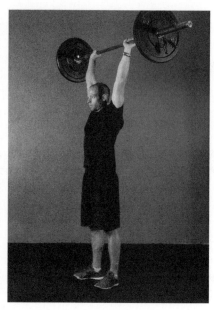

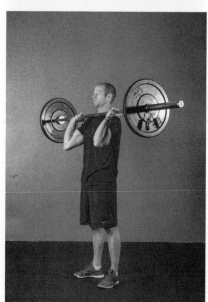

PUSH JERK

Stand with feet shoulder-width apart, weight racked on front of shoulder » Dip knees and drive weights upward, extending legs for power » Dip knees again to move under the bar » Lock out arms and return to standing position with weights overhead

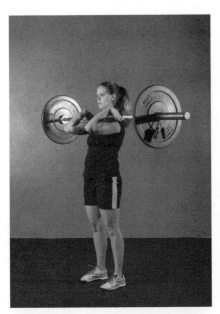
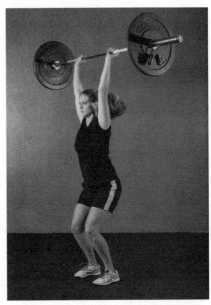
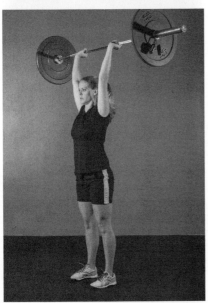

PUSH PRESS

Stand with feet shoulder-width apart, weight racked on front of shoulder **»** Dip knees and drive weights upward **»** Straighten legs and hold weights overhead

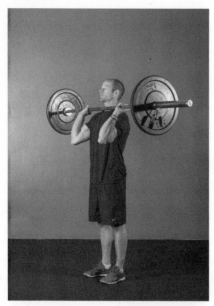
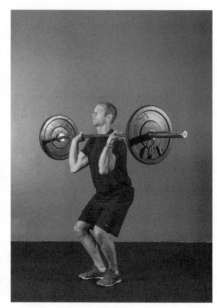
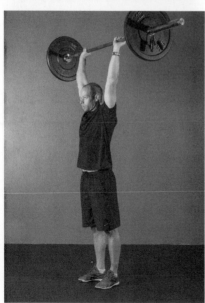

RING DIP

Press up into full extension ❯❯ Dip down with rings close to the body ❯❯ Repeat, bending at the elbows to lower yourself and then straightening them to again press upward

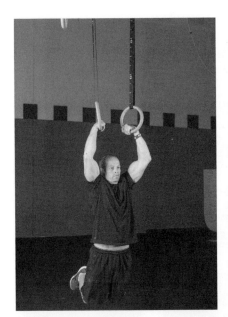
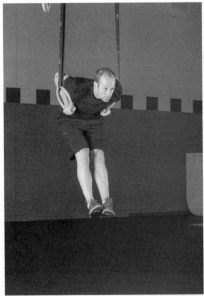

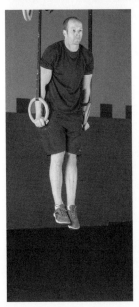
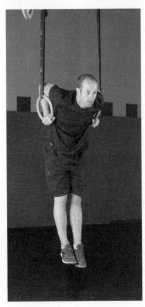
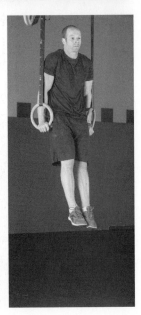

ROPE CLIMB

Pinch the rope between the feet as in the photo » Grasp as far up the rope as possible with both hands » Release the pinch and raise knees and feet as high up the rope as possible and re-establish the foothold » Then move up the rope by extending the legs (rather than pulling up with the arms) » Continue until you reach the top of the rope

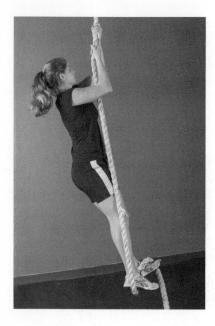

SNATCH

With feet shoulder-width apart, grip bar from the ground » Keeping weights close to the body, with knees still bent, drive bar upward » Squat beneath the bar and lock out the arms overhead » Assume full standing position

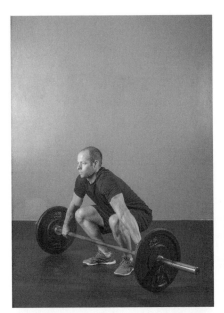

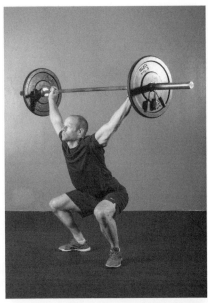

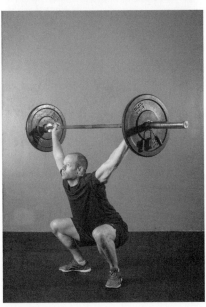

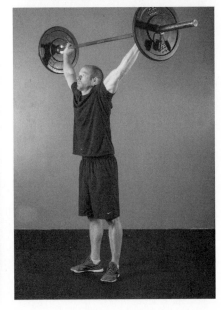

THRUSTER

With bar racked on front shoulders, perform a front squat **»** At completion of squat, use momentum to do a push press

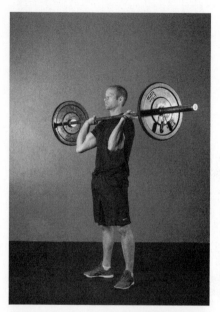 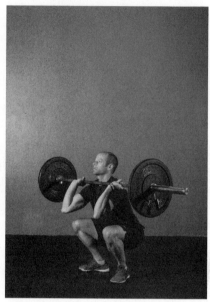

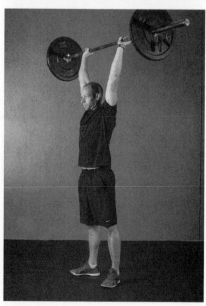

WALL BALL

From standing position, hold the medicine ball so that it touches the chin **»** Descend into a full squat and then drive upward with power from hips **»** Thrust ball to target on wall **»** Catch ball and descend back into squat

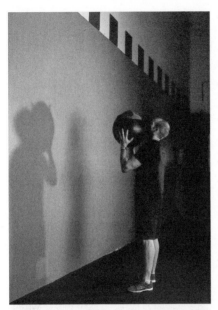 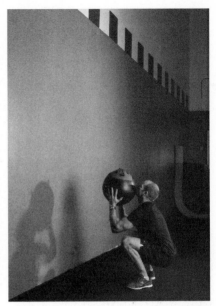

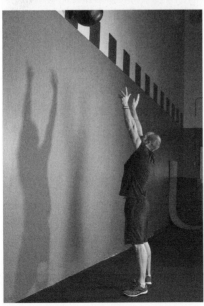